D0795556

NOT YOUR MOTHER'S
MEATLOAF

A Sex Education Comic Book

EDITED BY SAIYA MILLER & LIZA BLEY

SOFT SKULL PRESS

An imprint of COUNTERPOINT

BERKELEY

This book is a work of fiction. Names, characters, places, and incidents
either are products of the author's imagination or are used fictitiously.
Any resemblance to actual events or locales or persons, living or dead,
is entirely coincidental.

Library of Congress Cataloging-in-Publication Data is available.
ISBN 978-1-59376-517-0

Cover design by BriarMade
Interior design by Domini Dragoone

SOFT SKULL PRESS
An imprint of COUNTERPOINT
1919 Fifth Street
Berkeley, CA 94710
www.softskull.com
www.counterpointpress.com

Printed in the United States of America
Distributed by Publishers Group West

10 9 8 7 6 5 4 3 2 1

This book is dedicated to anyone
who has a story to tell.

CONTENTS

Chapter One: Beginnings

Chapter Two: Bodies

Chapter Three: Health

Chapter Four: Identity

Chapter Five: Age

Chapter Six: Endings

Chapter Seven: Personal Best

FOREWORD

There's something about *Not Your Mother's Meatloaf* that tears at your heart, in a good way. The stories are beyond honest; they reach out for your understanding. Even better, they broaden your respect for the many ways sexuality forms an individual. An older reader—someone past menopause, for instance—will gain a new appreciation of the complexities of the sexual minefields (a.k.a. opportunities) out there. The younger reader will feel comforted by knowing he or she is not alone. Not everyone will like every story. If this happens to you, just open yourself to a new perspective. Or just turn the page.

A couple of generations ago, I collaborated on an underground comic called *Tits & Clits*. Our idea was to do something radical based on "sex from a woman's point of view." This meant talking about birth control, abortion, menstrual blood, odors, wet spots, men, etc. In 1972, people found this topic unromantic, if not disgusting. We thought our stories were funny and feminist. GLBT awareness was beyond us at that time. It is gratifying to see that, after a lot of righteous criticism, our views have become part of a long-awaited and massive movement to open up sex for intelligent discussion.

The use of graphic narrative, comics, is finding its solid place in telling grown-up stories. Text, enhanced and illuminated by drawing, can transform a mere learning experience into something more personal, something memorable to the reader.

—Joyce Farmer
May 2013

INTRODUCTION

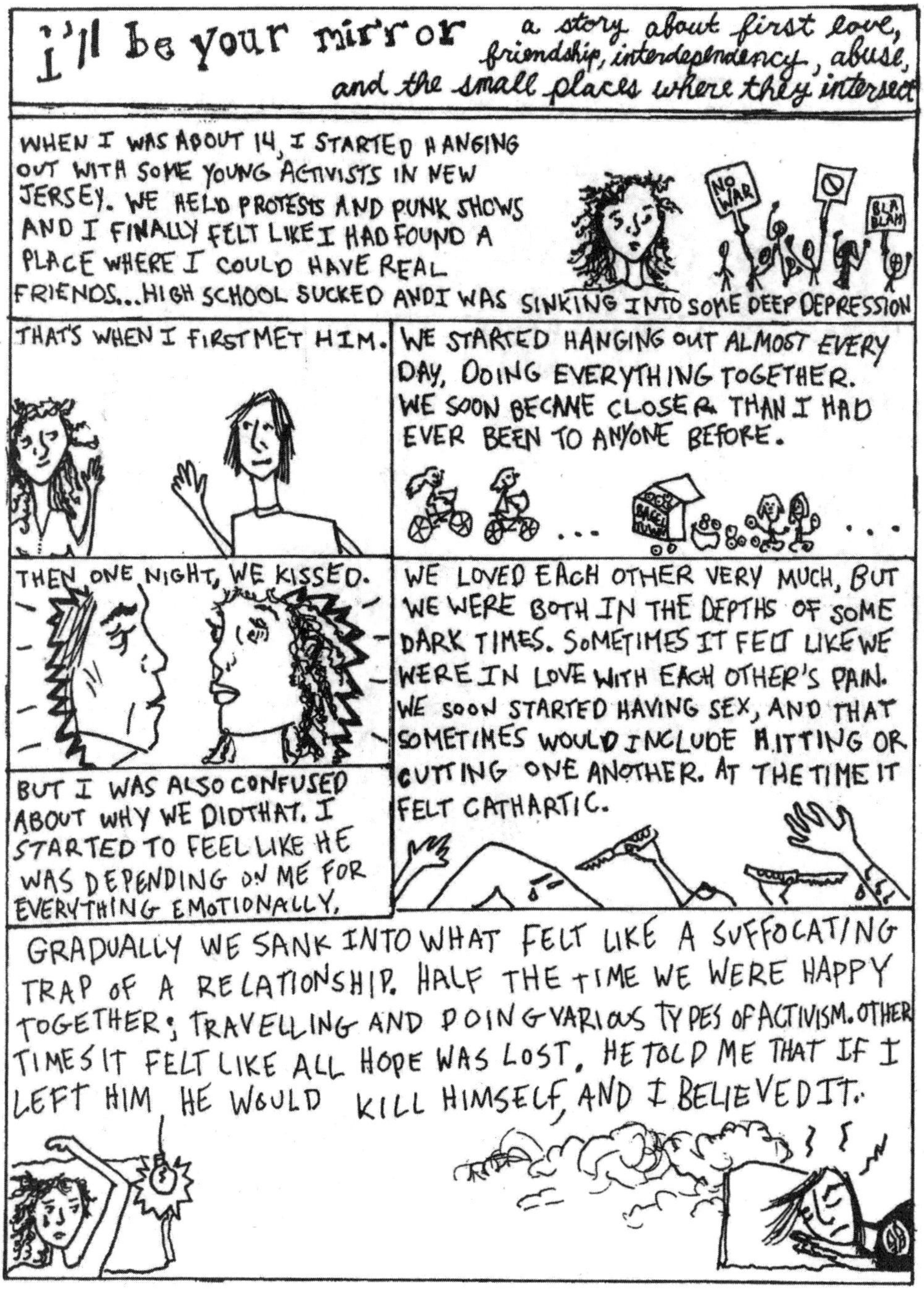
i'll be your mirror
a story about first love, friendship, interdependency, abuse, and the small places where they intersect
WHEN I WAS ABOUT 14, I STARTED HANGING OUT WITH SOME YOUNG ACTIVISTS IN NEW JERSEY. WE HELD PROTESTS AND PUNK SHOWS AND I FINALLY FELT LIKE I HAD FOUND A PLACE WHERE I COULD HAVE REAL FRIENDS... HIGH SCHOOL SUCKED AND I WAS SINKING INTO SOME DEEP DEPRESSION
NO WAR
BLA BLAH
THAT'S WHEN I FIRST MET HIM.
WE STARTED HANGING OUT ALMOST EVERY DAY, DOING EVERYTHING TOGETHER. WE SOON BECAME CLOSER THAN I HAD EVER BEEN TO ANYONE BEFORE.
THEN ONE NIGHT, WE KISSED.
WE LOVED EACH OTHER VERY MUCH, BUT WE WERE BOTH IN THE DEPTHS OF SOME DARK TIMES. SOMETIMES IT FELT LIKE WE WERE IN LOVE WITH EACH OTHER'S PAIN. WE SOON STARTED HAVING SEX, AND THAT SOMETIMES WOULD INCLUDE HITTING OR CUTTING ONE ANOTHER. AT THE TIME IT FELT CATHARTIC.
BUT I WAS ALSO CONFUSED ABOUT WHY WE DID THAT. I STARTED TO FEEL LIKE HE WAS DEPENDING ON ME FOR EVERYTHING EMOTIONALLY.
GRADUALLY WE SANK INTO WHAT FELT LIKE A SUFFOCATING TRAP OF A RELATIONSHIP. HALF THE TIME WE WERE HAPPY TOGETHER; TRAVELLING AND DOING VARIOUS TYPES OF ACTIVISM. OTHER TIMES IT FELT LIKE ALL HOPE WAS LOST. HE TOLD ME THAT IF I LEFT HIM HE WOULD KILL HIMSELF, AND I BELIEVED IT.

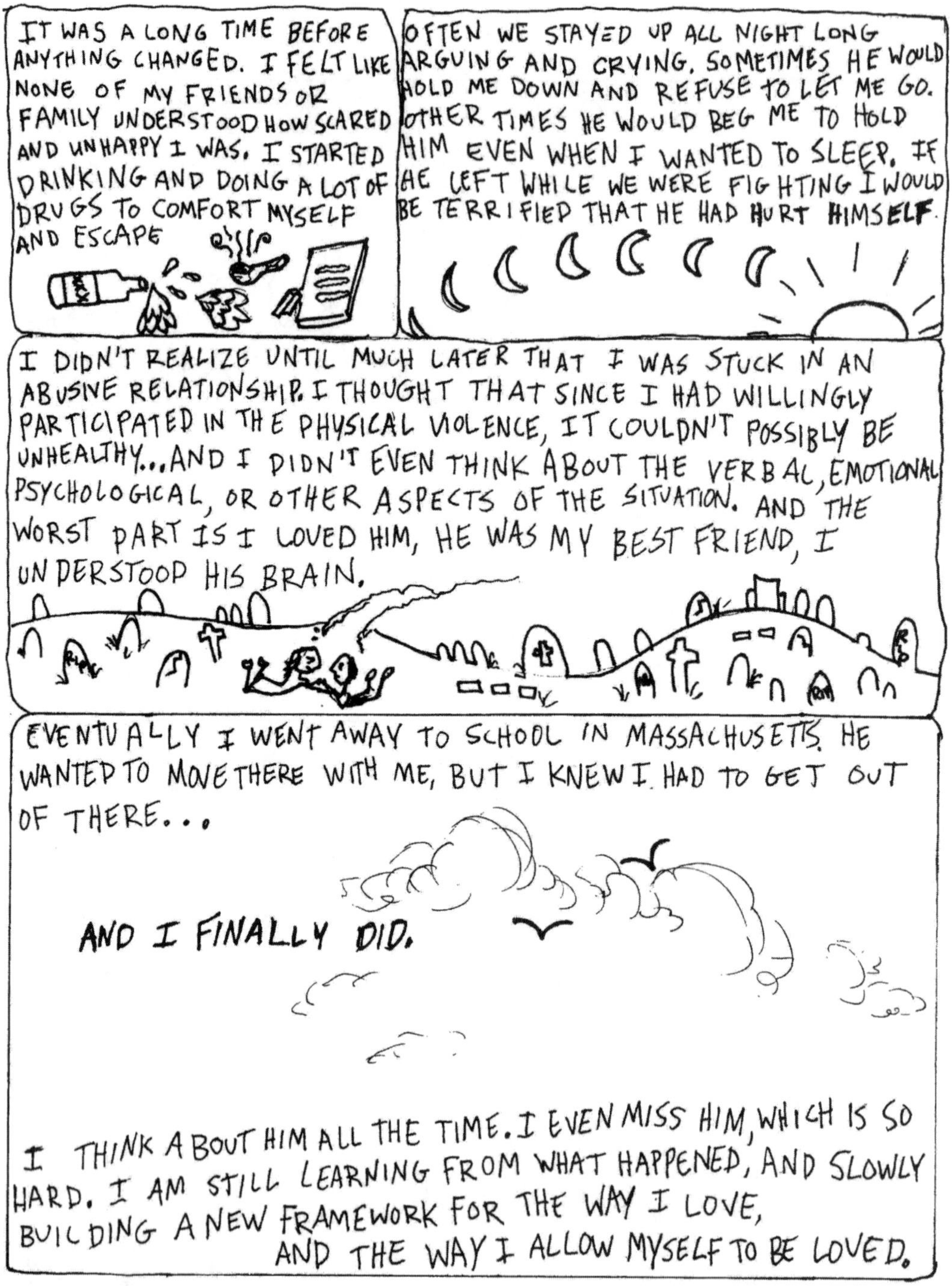
IT WAS A LONG TIME BEFORE ANYTHING CHANGED. I FELT LIKE NONE OF MY FRIENDS OR FAMILY UNDERSTOOD HOW SCARED AND UNHAPPY I WAS. I STARTED DRINKING AND DOING A LOT OF DRUGS TO COMFORT MYSELF AND ESCAPE
OFTEN WE STAYED UP ALL NIGHT LONG ARGUING AND CRYING. SOMETIMES HE WOULD HOLD ME DOWN AND REFUSE TO LET ME GO. OTHER TIMES HE WOULD BEG ME TO HOLD HIM EVEN WHEN I WANTED TO SLEEP. IF HE LEFT WHILE WE WERE FIGHTING I WOULD BE TERRIFIED THAT HE HAD HURT HIMSELF.
I DIDN'T REALIZE UNTIL MUCH LATER THAT I WAS STUCK IN AN ABUSIVE RELATIONSHIP. I THOUGHT THAT SINCE I HAD WILLINGLY PARTICIPATED IN THE PHYSICAL VIOLENCE, IT COULDN'T POSSIBLY BE UNHEALTHY...AND I DIDN'T EVEN THINK ABOUT THE VERBAL, EMOTIONAL PSYCHOLOGICAL, OR OTHER ASPECTS OF THE SITUATION. AND THE WORST PART IS I LOVED HIM, HE WAS MY BEST FRIEND, I UNDERSTOOD HIS BRAIN.
EVENTUALLY I WENT AWAY TO SCHOOL IN MASSACHUSETTS. HE WANTED TO MOVE THERE WITH ME, BUT I KNEW I HAD TO GET OUT OF THERE...
AND I FINALLY DID.
I THINK ABOUT HIM ALL THE TIME. I EVEN MISS HIM, WHICH IS SO HARD. I AM STILL LEARNING FROM WHAT HAPPENED, AND SLOWLY BUILDING A NEW FRAMEWORK FOR THE WAY I LOVE, AND THE WAY I ALLOW MYSELF TO BE LOVED.

SAIYA

Life started getting better, and for the moment I could ignore my past troubles, getting a break from the pervasive sadness. I had moved away from home, out of my parents' house, and I was starting to feel like a person with a life of her own. I had new friends, a new relationship, a new room—a new life—and it felt like a fresh start.

During the years before I moved away, I had a cold strength. I was fearless and coolheaded, so much so that people at school called me "ice queen." And it was true: I was cold because I had to be. If I seemed controlled, everyone would believe I was doing fine. I even believed myself sometimes.

This didn't last long. The icy layer was slowly cracking and melting away, and the new sprouts that shot up were angry and twisted. The feelings were messy and out of control, but they were warm.

Of course, the demons came anyway, showing up at times when I was weak or tired or homesick. They kept creeping back in all kinds of different ways. I would have paralyzing panic attacks, or I would space out and pick at a scab or pull my hair for what felt like an hour, and when I came to, I would be exhausted.

I had moments of uncontrollable rage. One day in my literature class, another student defended a male character in a book who had beaten his wife. Suppressing an urge to leap across the table, I tried to say something insightful and pointed, thinking I could control my anger long enough to change his mind. Instead my words quaked and shook and I found myself rising from my chair, storming out of the class, and running to the woods behind the building to shake and cry. I had never cried this way. I was surprised by how completely uncontrollable it was.

Years later, I would freeze up and space out during sex. I couldn't express emotion or even feel my body during these times. My inside self had taken a step back, leaving me just out of reach, a husk whose shoulder I watched over. I was aware of the change yet unable to break out of its iron grip.

I found I could not process the past. There was so much I needed to slog through, so many complicated things had happened, and I was still reeling from it all. I knew I would need to talk about it, but I needed a tangible way to unravel the confusion. It felt like another version of the relationship itself; I had known perfectly well that I was stuck and that it was abusive, but I could not escape until I had an excuse to move away.

Before I could move on, I needed to look further back.

LIZA

When I was growing up in Southern California, two of my playmates, a brother-and-sister duo, lived a couple of houses down. One afternoon when I was about six years old, the three of us played house. In our game of house there would be two parents and one child. We all knew, even in pretend, that a brother and sister could not be parents together, and it did not even cross our minds to pretend that two girls were the parents. This left only one option: I was the mother and the brother was the father. With our roles set, it was time for the parents to have sex.

In anticipation, my pretend husband and I took off our clothes and underwear. We got under the covers and rolled around over and under each other, like pigs in a blanket, while our pretend child played quietly on the floor. Sex was pretty fun, but after it was over, I felt guilty. This was not a typical game of house. Being naked felt wrong. Sex was reserved for adults, not six-year-olds.

Sometime later, my family and some of my parents' friends were eating lunch around our dining room table. Someone mentioned sex during the conversation. I whispered to my mother, "I had sex."

"What do you mean?" I came clean about my sex-having ways. She laughed, "Liza, that is not sex."

I was mortified: hot red cheeks. I hid in my bedroom until everyone left. My embarrassment stemmed from two places. First, all of the adults at that table knew that I had been naked and done sex. Second, and most horrible, they knew I had done the sex wrong and it didn't even count.

SAIYA

In elementary school I was prince of the tomboys. My hair was a frayed red rope and I had a gap in my front teeth so wide that I could shoot water through it, like my dad. Every day at recess I stomped past the Pokémon tree and the gossip bleachers and went to play soccer with the boys. I wore white undershirts with spaghetti straps and lace on the front, passed down from my mom to my sister to me. In fourth grade, something under those shirts seemed to be changing. I ignored my new chest for the year, and the year after, until sixth grade, when it became impossible to deny.

Everyone crossed a threshold once we got to middle school. My comrades, the boys who used to high-five me for my best jokes, were not to be trusted anymore.

While they puffed out their newfound chests and walked around like action figures, I adopted a sort of caved-in, folded stroll. I scoffed at the girls' attempts at hyper-femininity, hair straightened and faces frosted, yet I knew those things had their own powers and I should try them. But I still clung to my old style, and so emerged an odd combination of fashion elements, attempting to straddle the impossibly thin wall between genders.

By eighth grade I was at least outwardly reformed. Gel conditioner could dominate my uncontrollable hair, and when my mom and I went to the Salvation Army store, I scoured the place for clothes whose previous owner had gone on a shopping spree at the mall and then decided that the outfits were so last season. This act held up fairly well for the rest of that year, yet something felt deeply wrong. The farce was an airplane blanket; it managed to cover me but couldn't keep me warm. By the time I realized I would never *really* be a member of my soccer team, something snapped. I paced around our TV room, whispering under my breath, "I will reject that which rejects me!" I turned my shirts inside out and sewed patches onto them to hide the logos. I started playing guitar and staying up late in my room making weird paintings.

It was around this time that several formal discussions about sex came down from different authority figures. My mom explained sex patiently in the car and asked if I had any questions while I nervously gnawed on my seatbelt. Our health class also began giving us pathetic lessons in puberty, anatomy, and sex. It seemed like small potatoes compared to the slew of information scrawled on bathroom stalls and whispered in the halls and over lunch. Four of my friends and I experimented with posing and costumes in the basement of my house, taking pictures with a disposable camera that I believed to be so racy I waited years to develop them. We already knew as much as we possibly could about sex, so it seemed feeble that our teachers should tell us. When it came time to watch instructional videos about menstruation and pregnancy, or erections and wet dreams, boys and girls were herded into the gym and made to sit on opposite sides of a huge folding divider while our respective videos played. Everyone strained to hear the audio from the opposite side, and I wondered why we should only have to know about one set of bodily functions.

LIZA

From my earliest memories, an overwhelming amount of my life was focused on sex: daydreaming about sex, trying to define sex, watching sex, experimenting with sex, trying to have sex. It felt like pretend, a performance. I went from games of sex between my sheets to kissing classmates at recess. By the fifth grade I was in my first relationship with a boy. We kissed in the movie theater during *Starship Troopers* and I gave him a VHS copy of *Twister* for Christmas. From then on, I was hooked on the thrill of affection.

I moved from one elementary romance to another, orchestrated through AOL Instant Messenger and strategically exposed bra straps. Desperately, I tried to play the role. I wanted to be irresistible. I learned early to sacrifice parts of my identity in order to embody the feminine.

SAIYA

In many ways I cannonballed into my sexuality. At summer camp, spin the bottle was the source of most of my first kisses, and I tried dating a few scrawny elfin boys. I only had a brief period of time where it felt carefree and experimental.

My first real relationship felt fundamentally different from those previous ventures. He was four years older than I was, but somehow seemed younger, strange and quiet and angry behind long dark hair. There was something we got about each other, and we soon created a fortress around this newfound secret. I would sing a Nico song to him, "I'll be your mirror, reflect what you are, in case you don't know. I'll be the wind, the rain, and the sunset, the light on your door to show that you're home. When you think the night has seen your mind, that inside you're twisted and unkind, let me stand to show that you are blind. Please put down your hands, 'cause I see you." The song rang true; I served as a reflection for him. I validated him. My own reflection came back distorted and cracked, rendering myself unrecognizable. The kissing, and later the sex, perpetuated our dark pact instead of celebrating the good things we shared. It was violent and strange. He noticed that I had been cutting myself and said he wanted to cut me, too. This became a ritual, until one night when he cut my leg a little too deeply and I had to bandage myself up. I was strangely numb. He wanted me to choke him, hit him, fight with him in bed. When I did, it was as if I were watching him hurt himself, and I was just helping him out.

At fifteen I started taking birth control pills, which made me feel depressed and tired. If I looked back on my education about sex and made a checklist of all the things I had been told were important, it would have looked like I was doing fine. Condoms? Birth control? Check. Consent? Check. Getting tested? Check. The mechanics of sex were easy, and I thought I understood the facts of life. I was following all of the instructions I had been given, so why did it feel wrong? Why was I still so sad?

There were many discrepancies between what I had been told about sex and what I had experienced at that point. I had been thoroughly instructed about the functions of the reproductive system, but I had very little idea of what to expect when it came to my heart and my mind. There was no chart, no map. My only reference was other people, whom I looked to for answers.

The problem wasn't that I had no one to talk to. I talked to a lot of people, with varying degrees of honesty, about how my life had felt before and how it felt now. I told a friend about some of the more violent times, and she listened patiently while holding my hand. I told my mom about how unhappy and stuck I had felt back in New Jersey, and she apologized for not doing more to help me. I whispered in the dark to my new love, trying to explain that my lapses into frozen silence were not his fault, that they were only the past coming back to visit.

It certainly helped to talk. It was a good first step. The problem was that my story felt disjointed; it had so many disconnected parts that I spit out randomly. I couldn't present a cohesive narrative. It was like throwing pieces of my story down a well and trying to hear them hit the bottom.

LIZA

Just like the little girl who was mortified about not knowing exactly what sex was, I am still embarrassed when I don't know all the answers to my own body's questions. After years of repressing my genuine emotions, it was a habit to be insincere. Compiling *Not Your Mother's Meatloaf* over the past five years has helped me remember the importance of confronting this shame. Reading other peoples' stories has a powerful influence on interpreting my own sexual experiences. Working with Saiya is just the icing on the cake.

SAIYA

When I met Liza in New York, she shared her idea of putting together a sex education comic book. I knew that I needed it more than anyone. I had talked about my past, stewed on it for many sleepless nights, and thought I had a good handle on what I needed to work through. The process of comic making gave me a new level of understanding about my own experience. When I created a comic, I had full control of both the visual and written aspects of my memories. I could tell the story plainly and truthfully. I was able to say small yet true things inside those boxes, and what was too complex to say, I could draw.

I carried the scars with me, and I knew that I had learned something valuable from my past. There was a life lesson that I had tapped into early, a lesson about the give and take of intimacy.

It is not uncommon for these comics to be confessional, to tell about something that has never been revealed. One artist described it as packing up a room full of secrets, putting them into boxes, and lining them up in a row. The sequential visualization of a story can make it more manageable. It offers a form in which to organize the chaos of memory.

In the winter of 2008 we began collecting stories. We would sit in a loose circle in Liza's room, some of us on the bed and some on the rug or in chairs, talking about ideas for comics. One girl was drawing in her notebook on the floor; somebody else made popcorn and was passing it around while chomping loudly.

A girl with a shy, pale face and fringed strawberry blonde hair said, "I have a story I could tell . . ." She tilted her head back and shook her bangs to one side with a twitch, and they fell right back to where they had been before. "But I can't draw it."

"How come?" asked Liza.

"No," she said, flicking her bangs away again, this time with a more intentional flick. "I really don't feel like I can draw it at all."

"Well, what is it about?" asked the girl sitting next to her.

"It's about the first time I went to the gynecologist, but it was really bad. I mean, it was a tough experience. He was, like, a bad doctor. But I definitely can't draw it, so I don't know."

Something lit up in the girl sitting to her left, who said cautiously, "Maybe I could draw it."

The first girl lowered her brow slightly. "Yeah, that would be alright with me, I think."

They agreed to meet the following week after class and work on the comic together. I thought about how hard it would be to trust someone with such a personal story. Then again, I was curious about the possibility of freeing each person, sharing the weight of trauma, and allowing the story to come to the surface. The artist had no story of her own at the moment, and the author could not portray her story in pictures. The artist wanted to draw, to help the author process the memory in the difficult act of retelling. There are many ways we can find to describe our experiences and shoulder them together.

Sometimes it takes more than one person to tell someone's story.

ARE YOU GUYS VIRGINS?
LIKE HAVE WE HAD SEX?
YEAH. I'M A VIRGIN.
WAIT, DOES THAT COUNT?
I THOUHT YOU WENT DOWN ON Alex.
SEX CAN BE A LOT OF DIFFERENT THINGS TO PEOPLE. ONE DEFINITION IS: ANY CONSENSUAL SEXUAL EXPERIENCE INVOLVING AT LEAST ONE PERSON, EVEN MASTURBATION. SO, HOW DO YOU LOSE YOUR VIRGINITY? WELL... IT'S UP TO YOU!

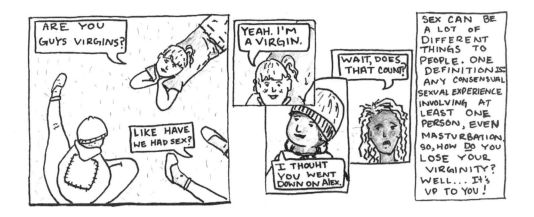

CHAPTER ONE:

BEGINNINGS

Children want to know about the beginning of things: how the world assembled itself around us, where we began. We want life to be told like a story, especially when it comes to making babies. We want to know how it all went down. Adults want us to understand, too, but only when we are ready. So, we are told a lot of creation myths. There are years of mystery, and even when some technical questions are answered, there is still so much left unsaid.

As we grow up, our questions about sex multiply. Instead of finding the few missing pieces, we discover more and more secrets. Like the Hydra sprouting heads, ten more questions come from the answer to one.

It is tempting to simplify the world of sex, love, and relationships, not only to be able to explain it to children, but to be able to reckon with it ourselves. We want to believe that there is order in the play of life: Act One is childhood and innocence; Act Two is teenage life and discovery; and by Act Three we are supposed to have a fully formed identity, and along with it, a road map to kissing, sex, and love. In reality, few of us ever live these plays. We have wildly different versions of the script, with notes scribbled in the margins, lines highlighted, and sections missing. The scripts beg for revisions. We experience first times and new beginnings over and over again. We sculpt ourselves like clay, constantly shifting and molding ourselves with each new exposure.

SAIYA

When my mom was pregnant with my little brother, my sister and I were given a book that set out to explain how babies are made. She was nine years old and I was four. We pored over the book, which was too big for our laps and had to be laid flat on the carpet. The story focused on a tall blonde woman and man who had apparently just gone shopping at the spandex and leg warmers store and were celebrating their new matching outfits by dancing and spooning at the beach. When you zoomed in on their hugs, though, science was at work. The diagrams on the pages that followed told small yet epic tales of adventure: sperm swimming toward an egg like the blown-away seeds of a dandelion in reverse; the egg on a voyage down the fallopian tube; a lima bean growing ears, legs, arms, and later a whole face. We understood that a baby was growing inside our mom, since it looked like she had swallowed a whole pumpkin. We began to understand how that egg turned into that baby. Something was missing, though, and it kept us awake at night wondering.

It was an essential detail of the story: how did the sperm get there in the first place? We flipped through the book searching for the answer. The story seemed to go straight from the beach scene to the pregnancy and birth. My sister thought she might know a clue, and flipped to the index at the back of the book to look up "penis." There it was! Listed at page 73. We flipped back, eagerly—page 70, page 71 . . . page 74? We were perplexed. The book had skipped two crucial pages, the only pages that we needed! Where were they? Had they forgotten to print them? We eventually accepted the book's mistake and moved on, still not really understanding the whole process.

My sister asked Mom how it really happened, skeptical that the baby in the book began to grow spontaneously. When we spit watermelon seeds off the back stoop in the summertime, we wondered if they would grow into vines in the backyard. Was it something like that? As usual, this conversation took place in the car, a place where we were afforded proximity without eye contact, but were also trapped. I nervously began gnawing on the seatbelt. My mother was clearly torn between being honest and being too honest. She compromised: "When a man and a woman are in love, they have a special . . . snuggle. The man puts his penis inside the woman's vagina. Then, a baby can be made." My seatbelt chewing intensified. It was terrifying, and also gross. "Snuggle" had been the wrong word.

Many years later, I returned to this baby book. Again I tried to look up pages 72 and 73, marveling over the missing link. This time, when I turned to the missing spot, I noticed something I had missed the first time around. If you peered very carefully between pages 71 and 74, into the crevice of the book's binding, there, lurking in between, was the smallest remaining strip of a page. My mouth fell open and I let out a shout of disbelief. It had not been a typo or a manufacturing mistake. Someone had deliberately cut out the page! I shook my head. It was time to find out the truth. Because this book was a bit outdated, it was hard to locate another copy in a bookstore or even on the Internet. Eventually I found one in the basement of a library in New York. Even though I had long understood everything I needed to know about how babies were usually made, I still flipped through this book with the same dangerous anticipation that I felt when I was four. And there, on page 72, was a full-color, heat-sensitized picture of an enormous erection. The technology they used to photograph it looked like the kind they used to find the monsters in the movie *Predator*. I laughed until I cried.

My sister and I asked my mom about it recently. She blamed our father.

"I know," she said, shaking her head. "Ridiculous." She gave out a little laugh. "The funny thing is, I was shown those same exact pictures as a child. Your grandma showed them to me, when they first came out in *Life* magazine. They were the first photographs ever taken in utero."

"That's kind of amazing, don't you think?" said my sister. "That they went and took pictures of space before they took a picture of a baby in a uterus."

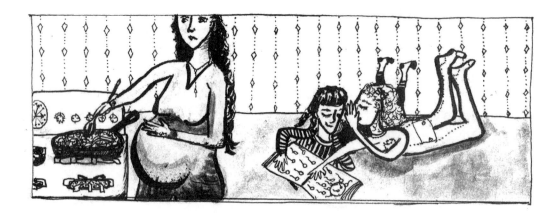

I agreed with her; it seemed like such crucial territory. It was incredible to see a picture of a baby in the womb, with its skin that the sun seemed to shine through, its fingers curled up into little glowing fists. But, then again, it was strange that my mother had learned about sex from the same blonde couple, had observed the same narrative about their beach date and mating dance, pillars holding up their model of reproduction for the rest of us to behold, generation after generation, for guidance.

LIZA

We were at the Royal Lee Bar and Grill, and I was 40 ounces deep. The Royal Lee let punk bands play a few times a month. Shows were all ages and the owners didn't stop us from drinking behind the building. Casey was thin and wore all black all the way down to his boots.

"Let's go to the alley," I said. I led the way. It was January and steam started rising from his shirt as soon as we got outside. He was wet with sweat from the pit. Our friends were just around the corner, drinking the beer we had stolen earlier that night. Before we got within eyeshot I grabbed his arm. He looked at me with an awkward, uneasy half-smile and I pushed him against the cold brick wall. I held his face and started to kiss him wildly. My hands moved from his face to his hips while my lips moved to his neck.

"Are you too drunk?"

"No!" I probably was.

Casey, recovering from the initial shock, started to clutch my waist and butt. He turned us around and pushed my body against the bricks. As he kissed me, he slipped his hand under my shirt and rubbed my naked back. We were a drunken mess of missed kisses and accidental stumbles, but perfect. We engaged hard for twenty minutes, until we heard the next band tuning up. I was sixteen, my lips were swollen, and this was the start of my healthiest relationship.

We both played the drums in punk bands and we both drank heavily. Before I dated Casey, I was in an emotionally abusive relationship. Because of this, it was difficult for me to be honest and vulnerable with him. In the beginning, Casey and I watched cartoons in his basement till one of us got drunk enough to make the first move. Alcohol was a crutch I used to dull the intimidation I felt. I did not believe Casey when he told me he liked me. When I was drunk, the relationship felt trivial. Alcohol masked my nervous fear of rejection and exposure, both physically and emotionally.

Our relationship progressed from heavy petting to hand jobs in the backseat of my minivan listening to Cock Sparrer on repeat. We became less dependent on malt liquor to initiate intimacy. We learned hand jobs were more pleasant with spit, Casey liked his testicles squeezed hard, and I enjoyed soft teasing on my clit, as opposed to rapid-fire friction. We moved on to oral sex, and what was once the climax was now just the foreplay. It was sloppy at first, but with our continued practice we gained the courage to communicate our likes and dislikes.

SAIYA

At some point, I became aware of a difference between learning about sex and learning about sexuality. There were physical technicalities and scientific formulas to explain the nuts and bolts of sex. If asked, these explanations were offered fairly freely. However, it was clear that sex was a multifaceted activity. It could exist in the context of procreation, but it could also exist for pleasure, and it could contribute to how a relationship might be defined. This was where sexuality branched off, becoming a total gray area.

Since my first real relationship was so troubled, I have had a lot of out-of-order firsts. My heart started out on the wrong foot or got out on the wrong side of the bed, and I have had to try to undo a lot of what I learned back then.

I had an experience when I first moved down to New York, when I was eighteen years old, that changed my outlook forever. I was transferring from one school to another, moving away from my beloved new friends and new boyfriend. I had cried on the drive down to the city, torn up knowing that I was doing the right thing for myself, but mourning the loss of the woods and the swimming holes and the people who had taught me how to be happy. The first weekend I was in the city, I wandered around alone for hours looking into store windows, turning to look at the passing people and dogs, my head feeling full and empty at the same time.

I ended up at a random bar, listening to bad karaoke and feeling increasingly hopeless, debating whether or not to just go home and watch movies. I was a little startled when a tiny but strong-looking woman approached me at the bar, introduced herself to me, and challenged me to a game of pool. When she talked she had a sideways smile that I liked. Before long, the game had been abandoned

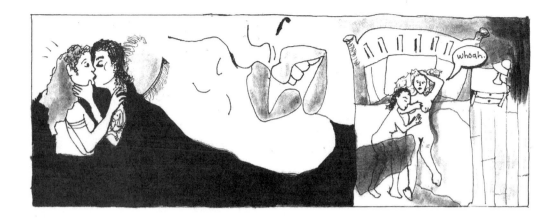

and I was sandwiched between her and the pool table. All of my frustrations and doubts melted away, and I followed her outside, down the block, and back to her house. Throughout the whole thing, we really communicated about what we wanted and what we were comfortable with. I learned that short-lived encounters can sometimes feel healthy. It was the first time I used consent with a stranger.

This felt like something to explore further. I began to sleep with lots of different types of people. Each person I encountered had a different way about them. Each had something new, an attitude that I could feel when we were together. I discovered that sex could feel good, could even be fun, could feel like love. Each person also had stories and history that stretched out behind them. I realized I needed to hear those stories, stories about things that really happened to people. I knew instinctively that only then could I tell my own.

LIZA

Casey said he was a virgin. I did not believe him. My previous partner lied about his virginity before we had sex, and I just assumed Casey would do the same thing. I often accused him of lying, even though he was always simplistically honest with me. We talked about having sex together a number of times. After a few months we decided to go for it.

I was not a virgin, but sex was still intimidating. It was scary to let Casey see me completely naked. I also worried that he would not enjoy having sex with me, that I would be horrible at it. We kissed and rubbed each other till he was very hard. He opened a condom and tried to put it on. It was backward and wouldn't roll down. We flipped it around and rolled it down his penis, not caring that the other side had already touched his tip and probably his pre-cum. We lay down on my bed, and he found my vagina with his fingers and then pushed his penis inside. Three slow thrusts later, he came. We got another condom and tried again. It was awesome.

We started having sex every time we saw each other. Once when my parents were away, I showed him how the water pressure from the bathtub faucet could make me orgasm. It turned him on to watch me cum. We went back to my room. As we were having sex, I ended up upside down, as if I were doing a handstand. Casey clutched my hips to steady me. We fucked for a while, me upside down and Casey right side up. As we experimented with different positions, laughter and excitement started replacing my feelings of vulnerability.

SAIYA

I had so much to learn, and I felt like a total rookie. My reflection was still hazy. I needed to investigate myself beyond the difference between having a bad boyfriend and having a good boyfriend. Back up north I had found someone I loved, whose love was strong and not fickle, but the world was wide and full of people, and the city showed me that every day. I had always felt older than my age, wise before my time, heavyhearted from what I had already seen. In the city I really felt young. I realized I was in a better place and I could start over, almost fresh, and try some different stuff. It was a time of exploration, my renaissance of firsts.

LIZA

That relationship born from stale beer and winter alleys remains the only one in which I felt truly safe and loved. We were always able to experiment with each other's bodies. In our last days we rented a motel room on Route 29. It had a nautical theme. We drank hard lemonade, I wore a sexy maid's costume, and he asked if he could slap me in the face with his hard cock. I said yes. I have never experienced the same free-falling trust with a sexual partner or felt as comfortable with my body next to another's again.

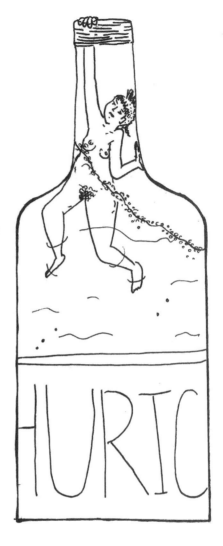

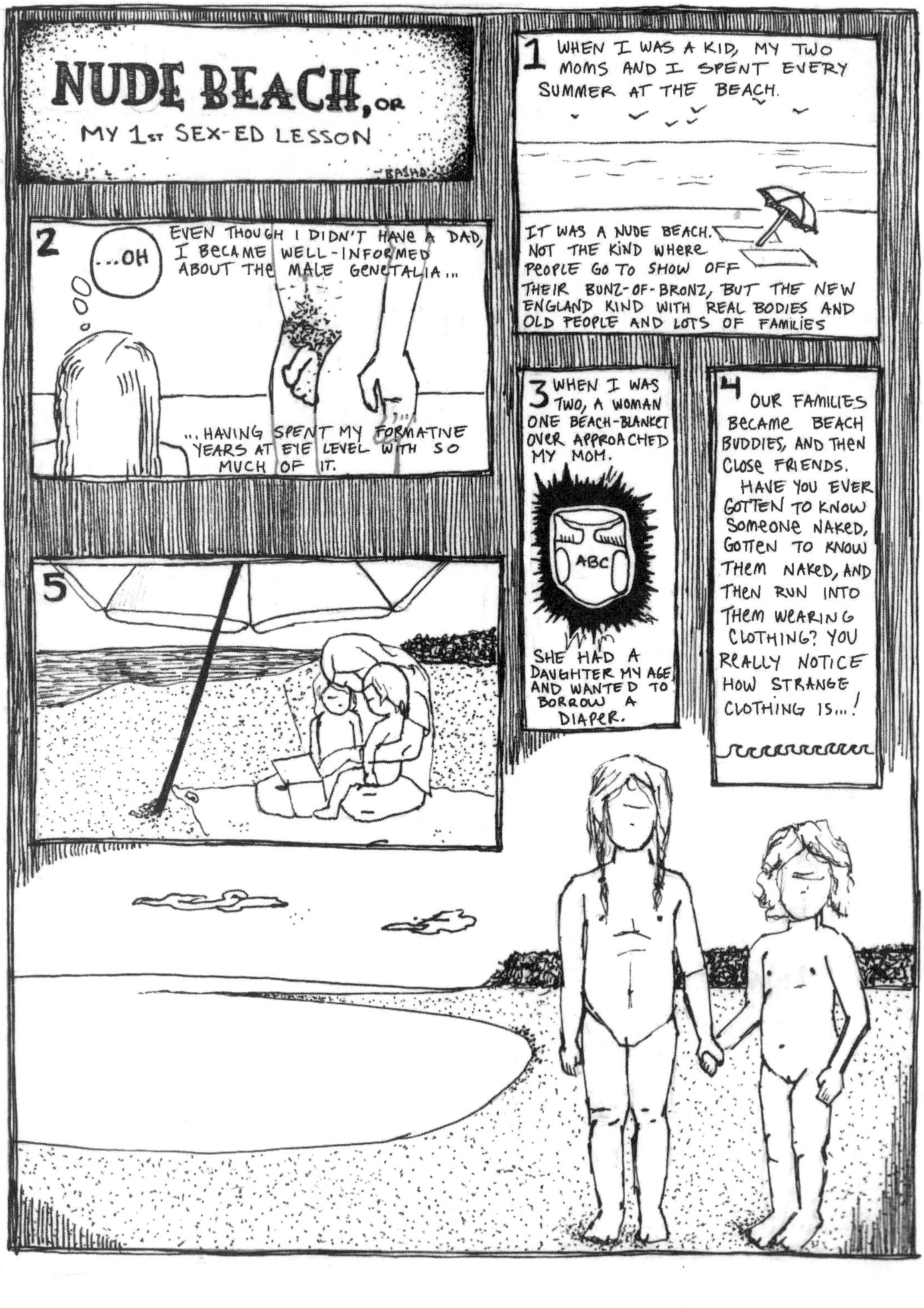
NUDE BEACH, OR
MY 1ST SEX-ED LESSON
-BASHA
1 WHEN I WAS A KID, MY TWO MOMS AND I SPENT EVERY SUMMER AT THE BEACH.
IT WAS A NUDE BEACH. NOT THE KIND WHERE PEOPLE GO TO SHOW OFF THEIR BUNZ-OF-BRONZ, BUT THE NEW ENGLAND KIND WITH REAL BODIES AND OLD PEOPLE AND LOTS OF FAMILIES
2 EVEN THOUGH I DIDN'T HAVE A DAD, I BECAME WELL-INFORMED ABOUT THE MALE GENETALIA...
...OH
...HAVING SPENT MY FORMATIVE YEARS AT EYE LEVEL WITH SO MUCH OF IT.
3 WHEN I WAS TWO, A WOMAN ONE BEACH-BLANKET OVER APPROACHED MY MOM.
ABC
SHE HAD A DAUGHTER MY AGE AND WANTED TO BORROW A DIAPER.
4 OUR FAMILIES BECAME BEACH BUDDIES, AND THEN CLOSE FRIENDS.
HAVE YOU EVER GOTTEN TO KNOW SOMEONE NAKED, GOTTEN TO KNOW THEM NAKED, AND THEN RUN INTO THEM WEARING CLOTHING? YOU REALLY NOTICE HOW STRANGE CLOTHING IS...!
5

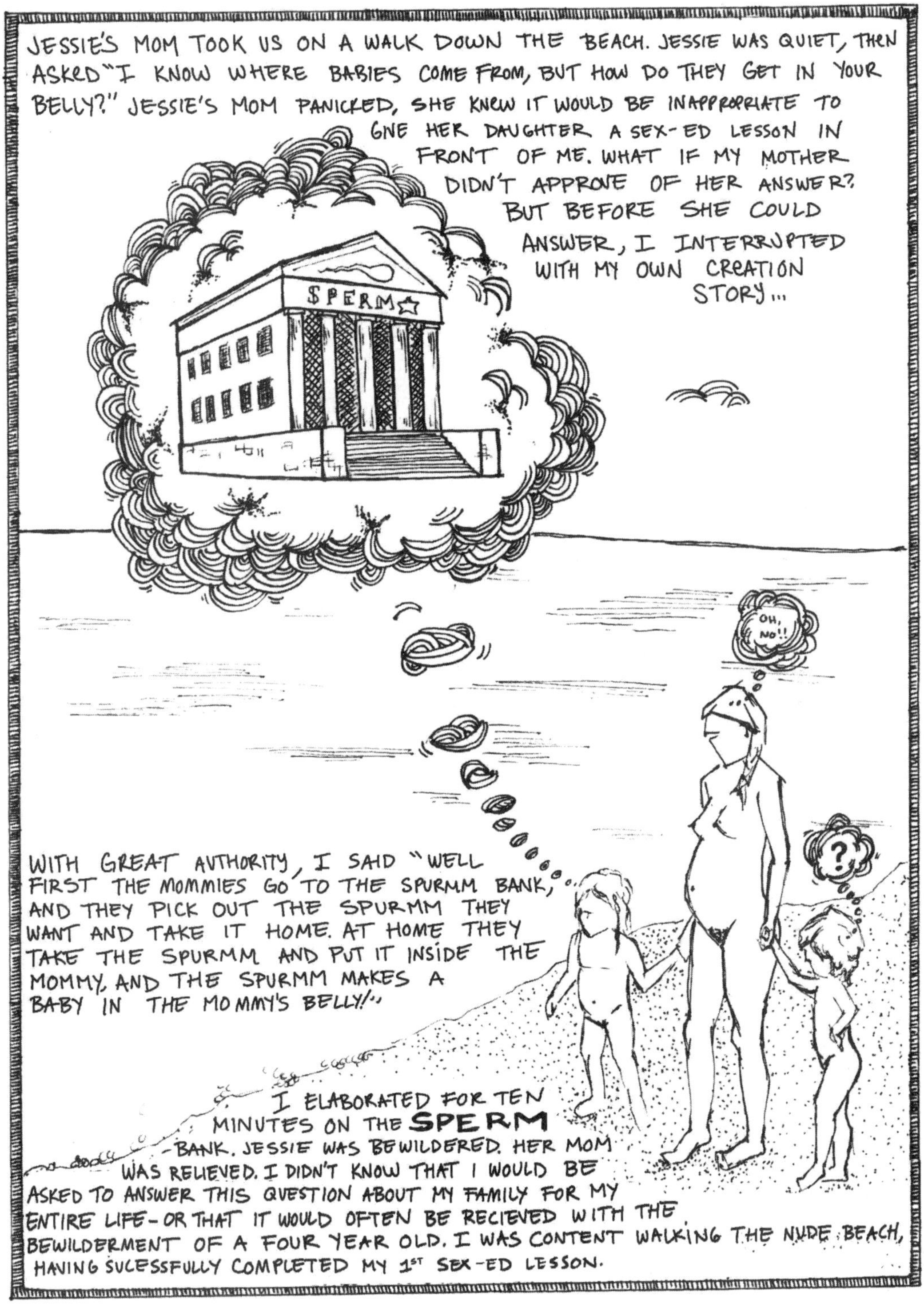
JESSIE'S MOM TOOK US ON A WALK DOWN THE BEACH. JESSIE WAS QUIET, THEN ASKED "I KNOW WHERE BABIES COME FROM, BUT HOW DO THEY GET IN YOUR BELLY?" JESSIE'S MOM PANICKED, SHE KNEW IT WOULD BE INAPPROPRIATE TO GIVE HER DAUGHTER A SEX-ED LESSON IN FRONT OF ME. WHAT IF MY MOTHER DIDN'T APPROVE OF HER ANSWER? BUT BEFORE SHE COULD ANSWER, I INTERRUPTED WITH MY OWN CREATION STORY...
SPERM
OH, NO!!
?
WITH GREAT AUTHORITY, I SAID "WELL FIRST THE MOMMIES GO TO THE SPURMM BANK, AND THEY PICK OUT THE SPURMM THEY WANT AND TAKE IT HOME. AT HOME THEY TAKE THE SPURMM AND PUT IT INSIDE THE MOMMY, AND THE SPURMM MAKES A BABY IN THE MOMMY'S BELLY!"
I ELABORATED FOR TEN MINUTES ON THE SPERM-BANK. JESSIE WAS BEWILDERED. HER MOM WAS RELIEVED. I DIDN'T KNOW THAT I WOULD BE ASKED TO ANSWER THIS QUESTION ABOUT MY FAMILY FOR MY ENTIRE LIFE - OR THAT IT WOULD OFTEN BE RECIEVED WITH THE BEWILDERMENT OF A FOUR YEAR OLD. I WAS CONTENT WALKING THE NUDE BEACH, HAVING SUCESSFULLY COMPLETED MY 1ST SEX-ED LESSON.

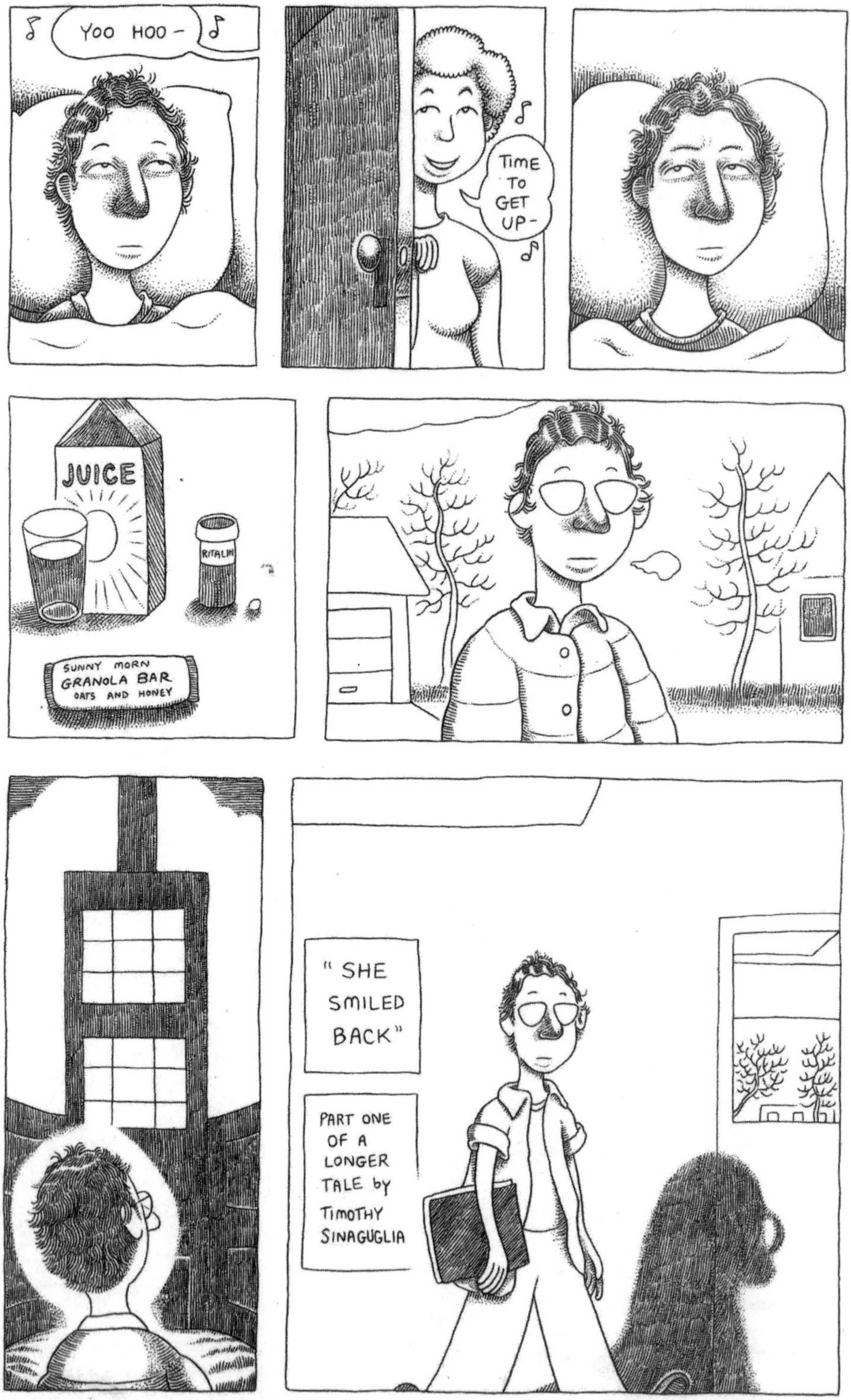
YOO HOO-
TIME TO GET UP-
JUICE
RITALIN
SUNNY MORN
GRANOLA BAR
OATS AND HONEY
" SHE SMILED BACK"
PART ONE OF A LONGER TALE by TIMOTHY SINAGUGLIA

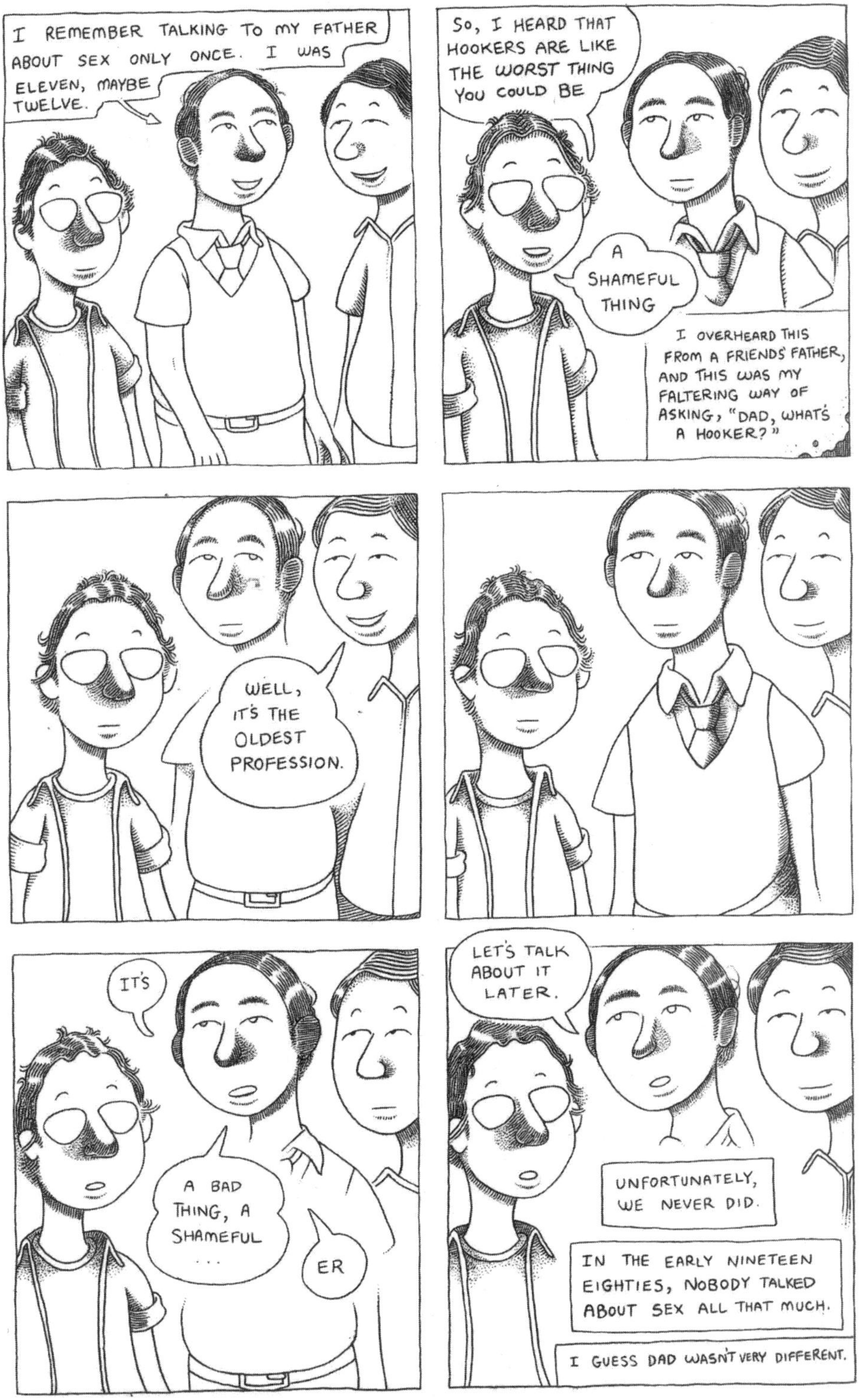
I REMEMBER TALKING TO MY FATHER ABOUT SEX ONLY ONCE. I WAS ELEVEN, MAYBE TWELVE.
So, I HEARD THAT HOOKERS ARE LIKE THE WORST THING YOU COULD BE
A SHAMEFUL THING
I OVERHEARD THIS FROM A FRIENDS' FATHER, AND THIS WAS MY FALTERING WAY OF ASKING, "DAD, WHAT'S A HOOKER?"
WELL, IT'S THE OLDEST PROFESSION.
IT'S
A BAD THING, A SHAMEFUL . . .
ER
LET'S TALK ABOUT IT LATER.
UNFORTUNATELY, WE NEVER DID.
IN THE EARLY NINETEEN EIGHTIES, NOBODY TALKED ABOUT SEX ALL THAT MUCH.
I GUESS DAD WASN'T VERY DIFFERENT.

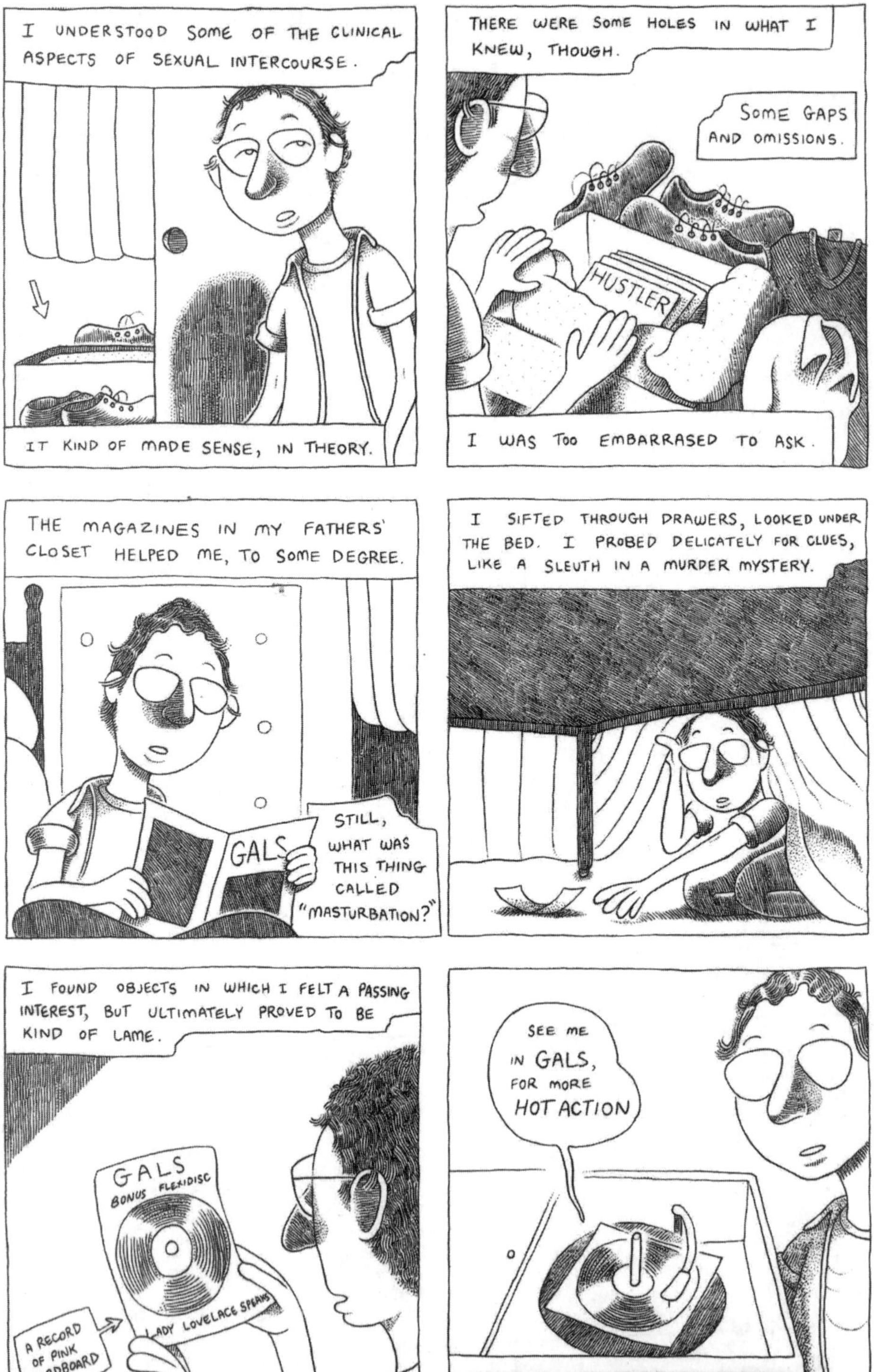
I UNDERSTOOD SOME OF THE CLINICAL ASPECTS OF SEXUAL INTERCOURSE.
IT KIND OF MADE SENSE, IN THEORY.
THERE WERE SOME HOLES IN WHAT I KNEW, THOUGH.
SOME GAPS AND OMISSIONS.
HUSTLER
I WAS TOO EMBARRASED TO ASK.
THE MAGAZINES IN MY FATHERS' CLOSET HELPED ME, TO SOME DEGREE.
GALS
STILL, WHAT WAS THIS THING CALLED "MASTURBATION?"
I SIFTED THROUGH DRAWERS, LOOKED UNDER THE BED. I PROBED DELICATELY FOR CLUES, LIKE A SLEUTH IN A MURDER MYSTERY.
I FOUND OBJECTS IN WHICH I FELT A PASSING INTEREST, BUT ULTIMATELY PROVED TO BE KIND OF LAME.
GALS
BONUS FLEXIDISC
LADY LOVELACE SPEAKS
A RECORD OF PINK CARDBOARD
SEE ME IN GALS, FOR MORE HOT ACTION

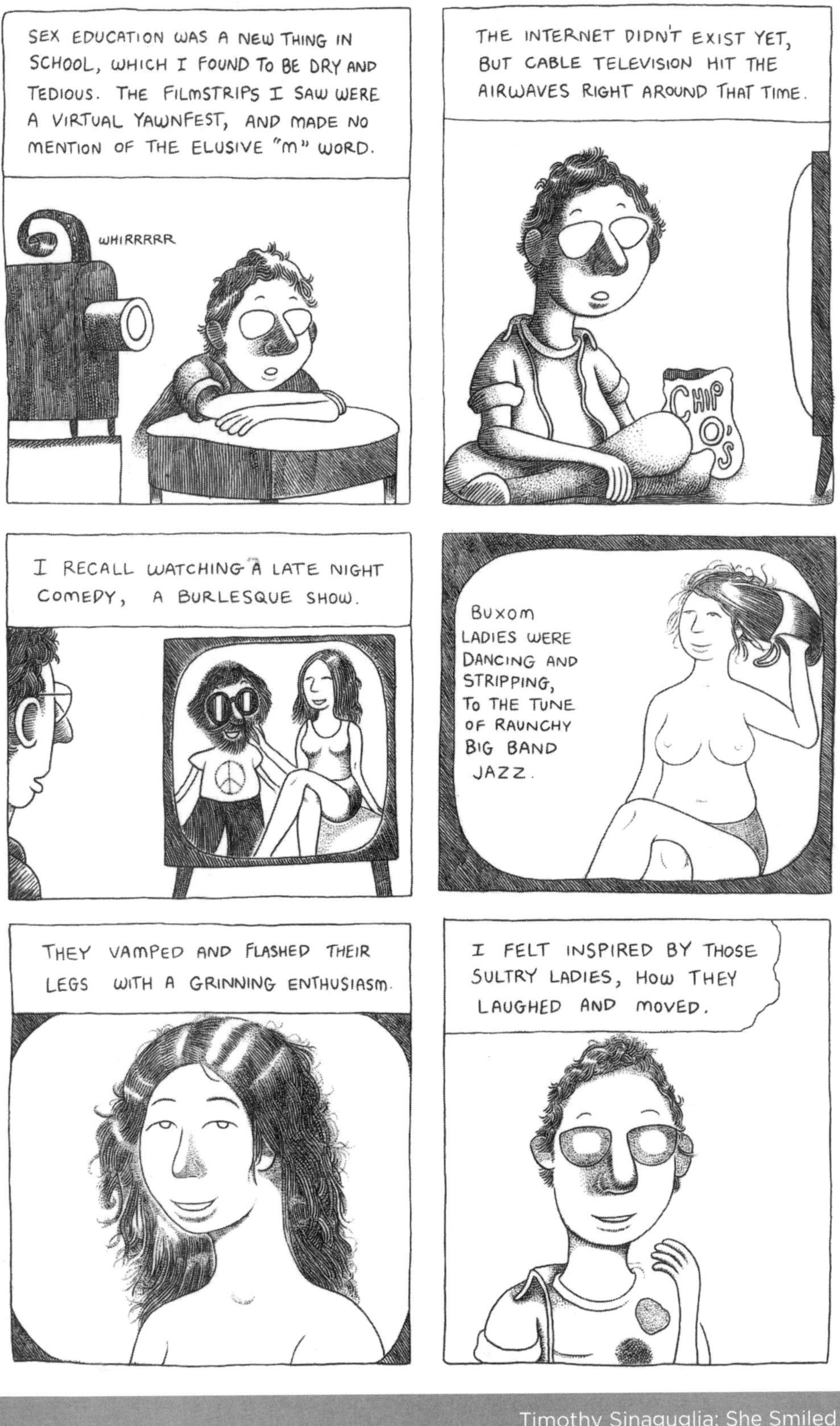
SEX EDUCATION WAS A NEW THING IN SCHOOL, WHICH I FOUND TO BE DRY AND TEDIOUS. THE FILMSTRIPS I SAW WERE A VIRTUAL YAWNFEST, AND MADE NO MENTION OF THE ELUSIVE "M" WORD.
WHIRRRRR
THE INTERNET DIDN'T EXIST YET, BUT CABLE TELEVISION HIT THE AIRWAVES RIGHT AROUND THAT TIME.
CHIP O'S
I RECALL WATCHING A LATE NIGHT COMEDY, A BURLESQUE SHOW.
BUXOM LADIES WERE DANCING AND STRIPPING, TO THE TUNE OF RAUNCHY BIG BAND JAZZ.
THEY VAMPED AND FLASHED THEIR LEGS WITH A GRINNING ENTHUSIASM.
I FELT INSPIRED BY THOSE SULTRY LADIES, HOW THEY LAUGHED AND MOVED.

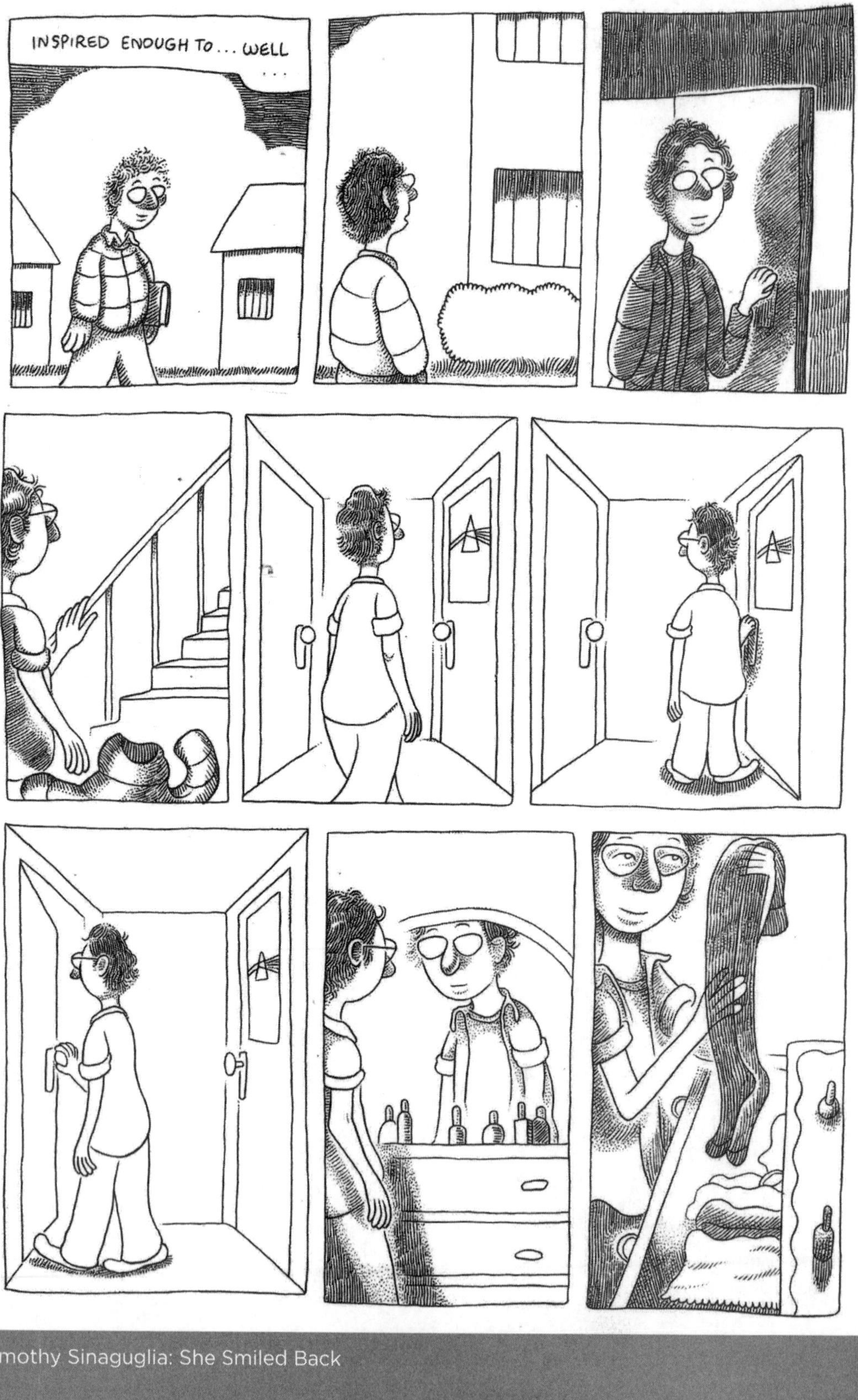
INSPIRED ENOUGH TO... WELL
...

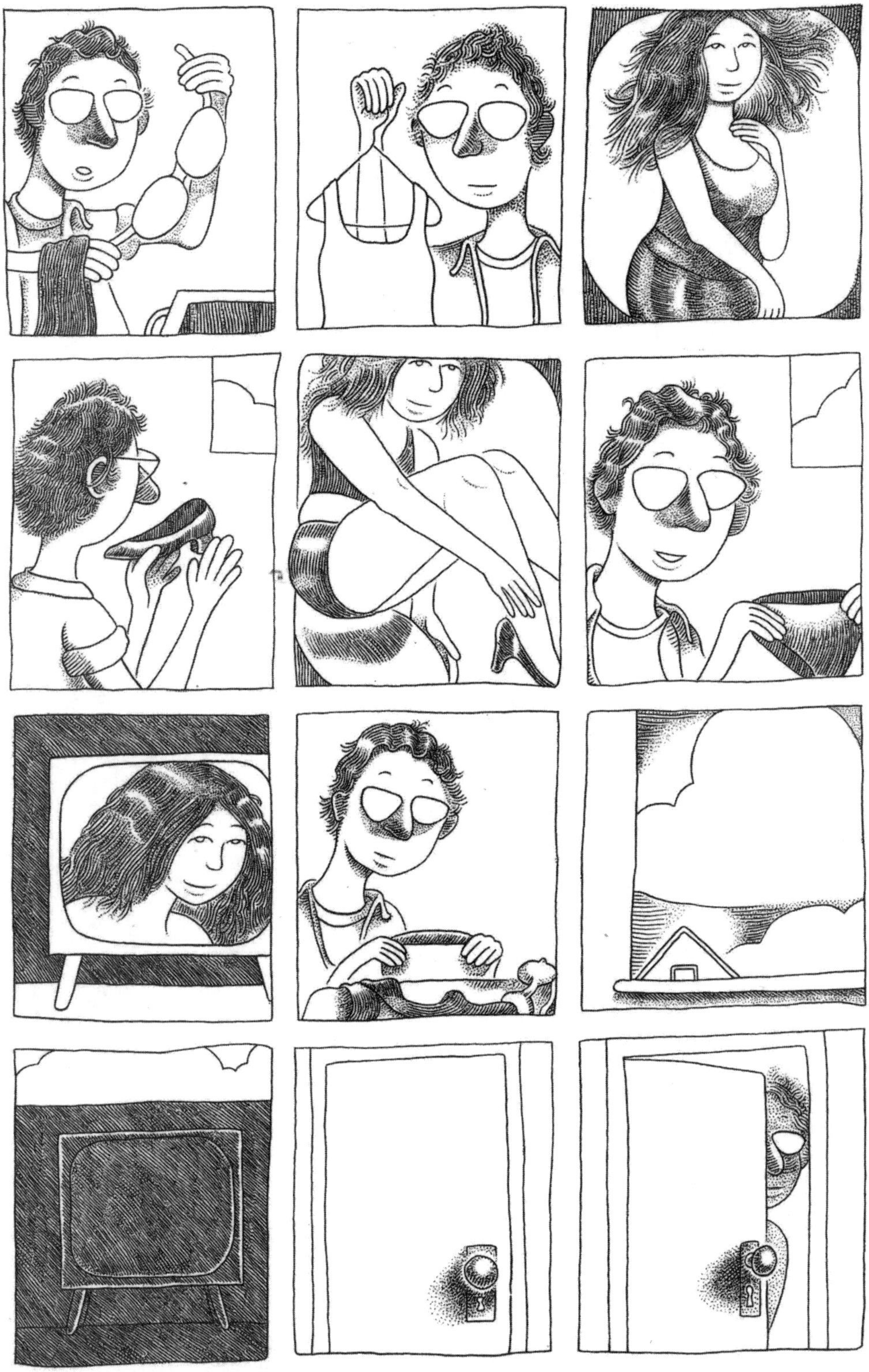

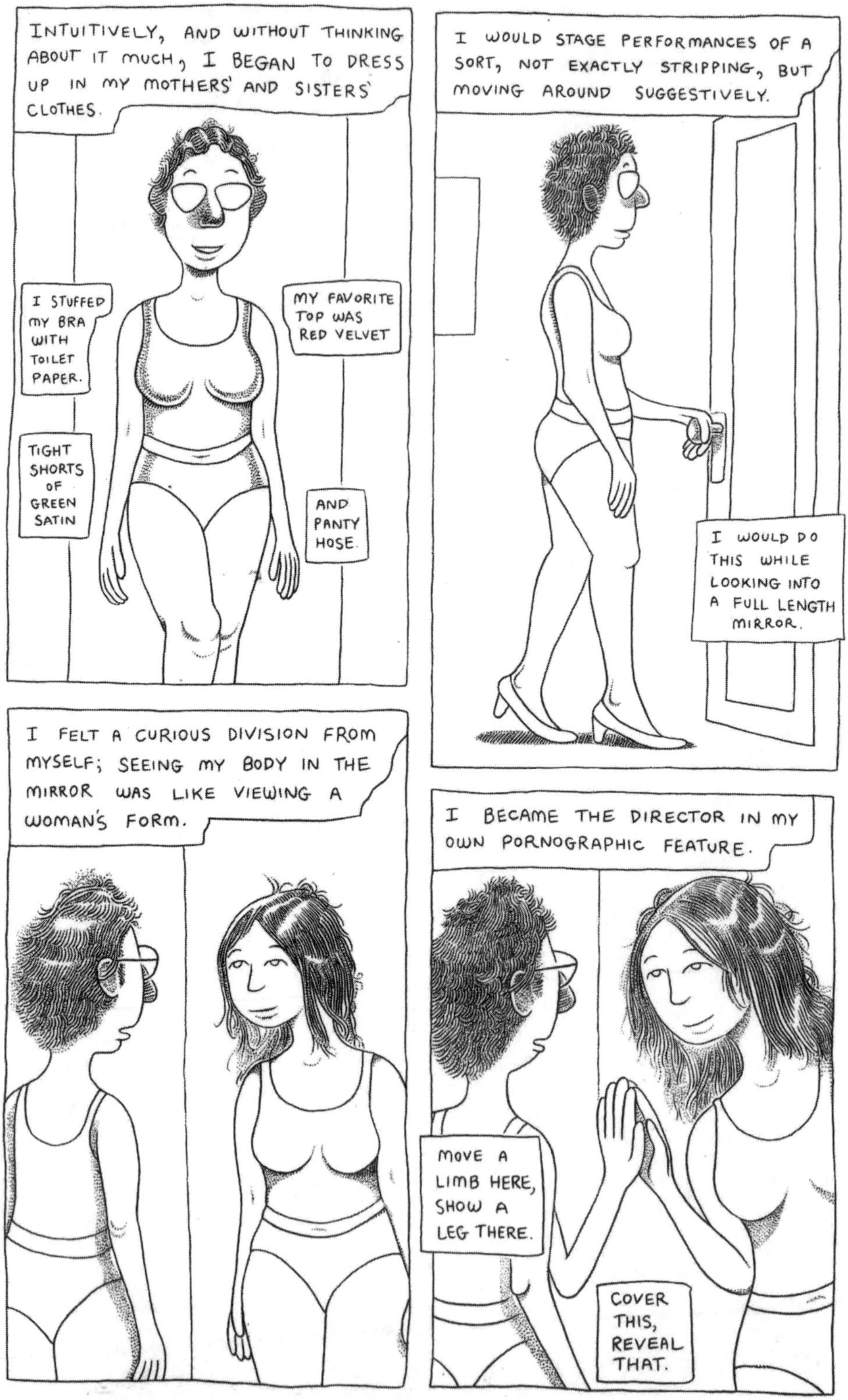
INTUITIVELY, AND WITHOUT THINKING ABOUT IT MUCH, I BEGAN TO DRESS UP IN MY MOTHERS' AND SISTERS' CLOTHES.
I STUFFED MY BRA WITH TOILET PAPER.
MY FAVORITE TOP WAS RED VELVET
TIGHT SHORTS OF GREEN SATIN
AND PANTY HOSE.
I WOULD STAGE PERFORMANCES OF A SORT, NOT EXACTLY STRIPPING, BUT MOVING AROUND SUGGESTIVELY.
I WOULD DO THIS WHILE LOOKING INTO A FULL LENGTH MIRROR.
I FELT A CURIOUS DIVISION FROM MYSELF; SEEING MY BODY IN THE MIRROR WAS LIKE VIEWING A WOMAN'S FORM.
I BECAME THE DIRECTOR IN MY OWN PORNOGRAPHIC FEATURE.
MOVE A LIMB HERE, SHOW A LEG THERE.
COVER THIS, REVEAL THAT.

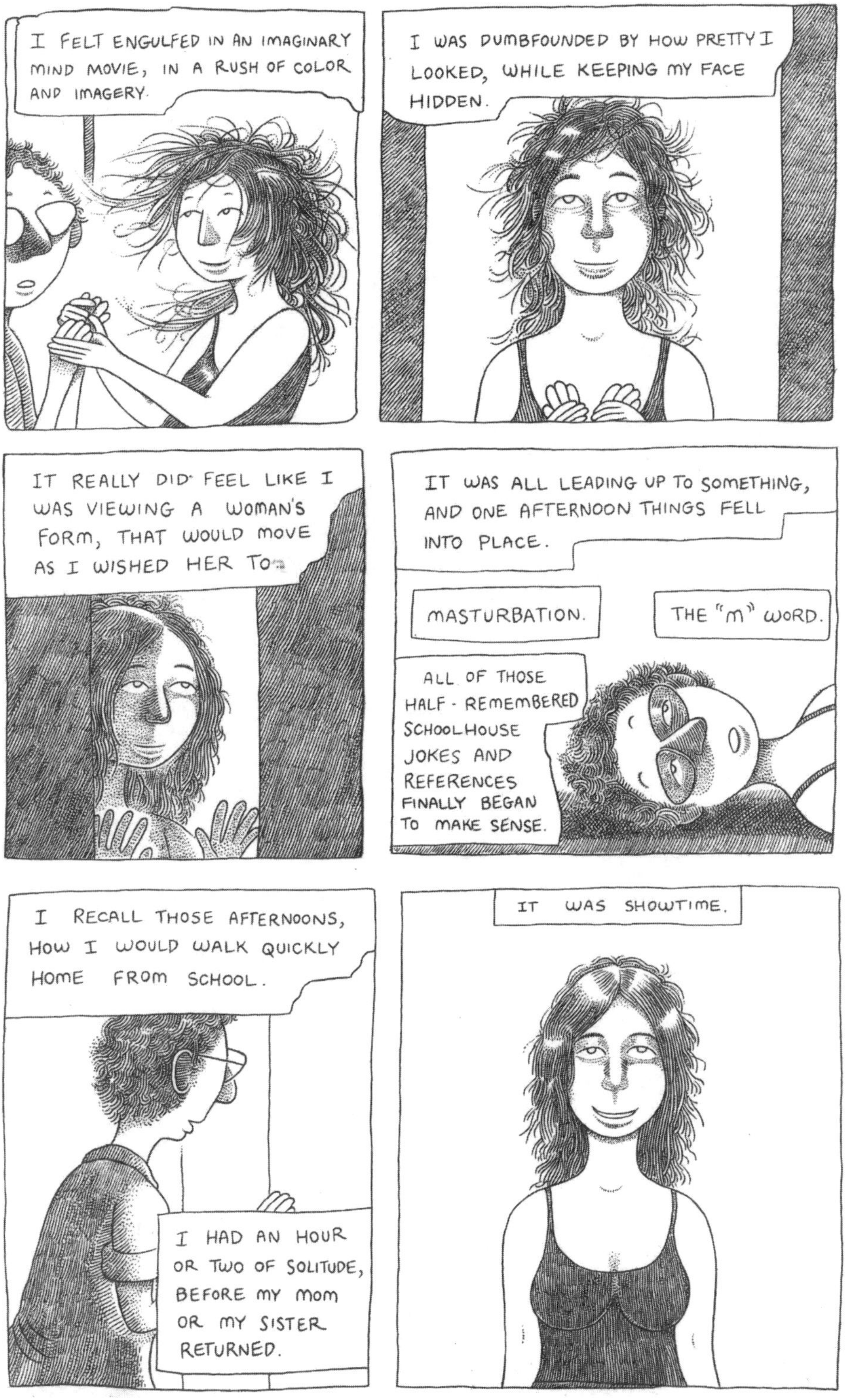
I FELT ENGULFED IN AN IMAGINARY MIND MOVIE, IN A RUSH OF COLOR AND IMAGERY.
I WAS DUMBFOUNDED BY HOW PRETTY I LOOKED, WHILE KEEPING MY FACE HIDDEN.
IT REALLY DID FEEL LIKE I WAS VIEWING A WOMAN'S FORM, THAT WOULD MOVE AS I WISHED HER TO.
IT WAS ALL LEADING UP TO SOMETHING, AND ONE AFTERNOON THINGS FELL INTO PLACE.
MASTURBATION.
THE "M" WORD.
ALL OF THOSE HALF-REMEMBERED SCHOOLHOUSE JOKES AND REFERENCES FINALLY BEGAN TO MAKE SENSE.
I RECALL THOSE AFTERNOONS, HOW I WOULD WALK QUICKLY HOME FROM SCHOOL.
I HAD AN HOUR OR TWO OF SOLITUDE, BEFORE MY MOM OR MY SISTER RETURNED.
IT WAS SHOWTIME.

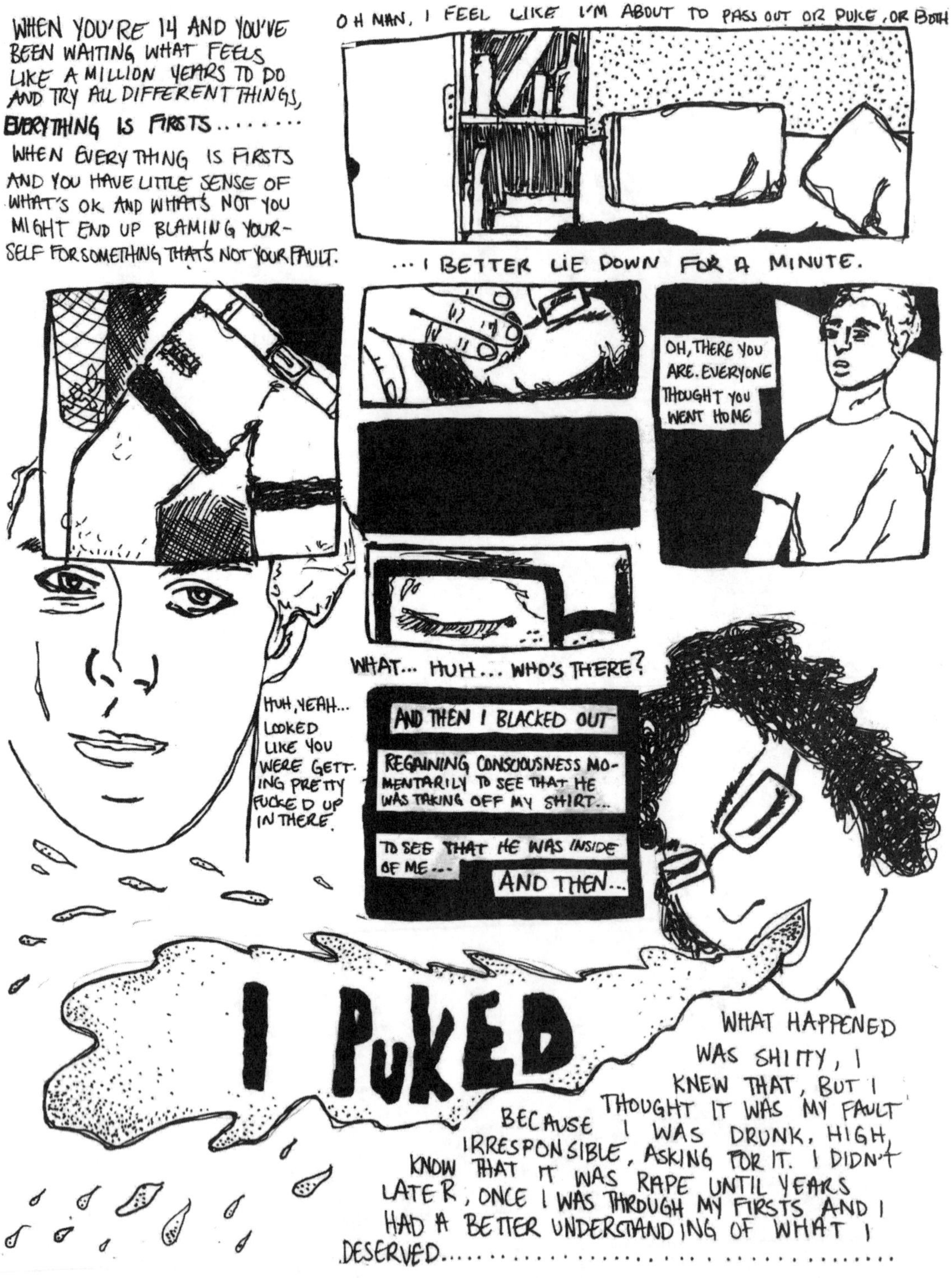
WHEN YOU'RE 14 AND YOU'VE BEEN WAITING WHAT FEELS LIKE A MILLION YEARS TO DO AND TRY ALL DIFFERENT THINGS,
EVERYTHING IS FIRSTS........
WHEN EVERYTHING IS FIRSTS AND YOU HAVE LITTLE SENSE OF WHAT'S OK AND WHAT'S NOT YOU MIGHT END UP BLAMING YOURSELF FOR SOMETHING THAT'S NOT YOUR FAULT.
OH MAN, I FEEL LIKE I'M ABOUT TO PASS OUT OR PUKE, OR BOTH
...I BETTER LIE DOWN FOR A MINUTE.
OH, THERE YOU ARE. EVERYONE THOUGHT YOU WENT HOME
HUH, YEAH... LOOKED LIKE YOU WERE GETTING PRETTY FUCKED UP IN THERE.
WHAT... HUH... WHO'S THERE?
AND THEN I BLACKED OUT
REGAINING CONSCIOUSNESS MOMENTARILY TO SEE THAT HE WAS TAKING OFF MY SHIRT...
TO SEE THAT HE WAS INSIDE OF ME...
AND THEN...
I PUKED
WHAT HAPPENED WAS SHITTY, I KNEW THAT, BUT I THOUGHT IT WAS MY FAULT BECAUSE I WAS DRUNK, HIGH, IRRESPONSIBLE, ASKING FOR IT. I DIDN'T KNOW THAT IT WAS RAPE UNTIL YEARS LATER, ONCE I WAS THROUGH MY FIRSTS AND I HAD A BETTER UNDERSTANDING OF WHAT I DESERVED......

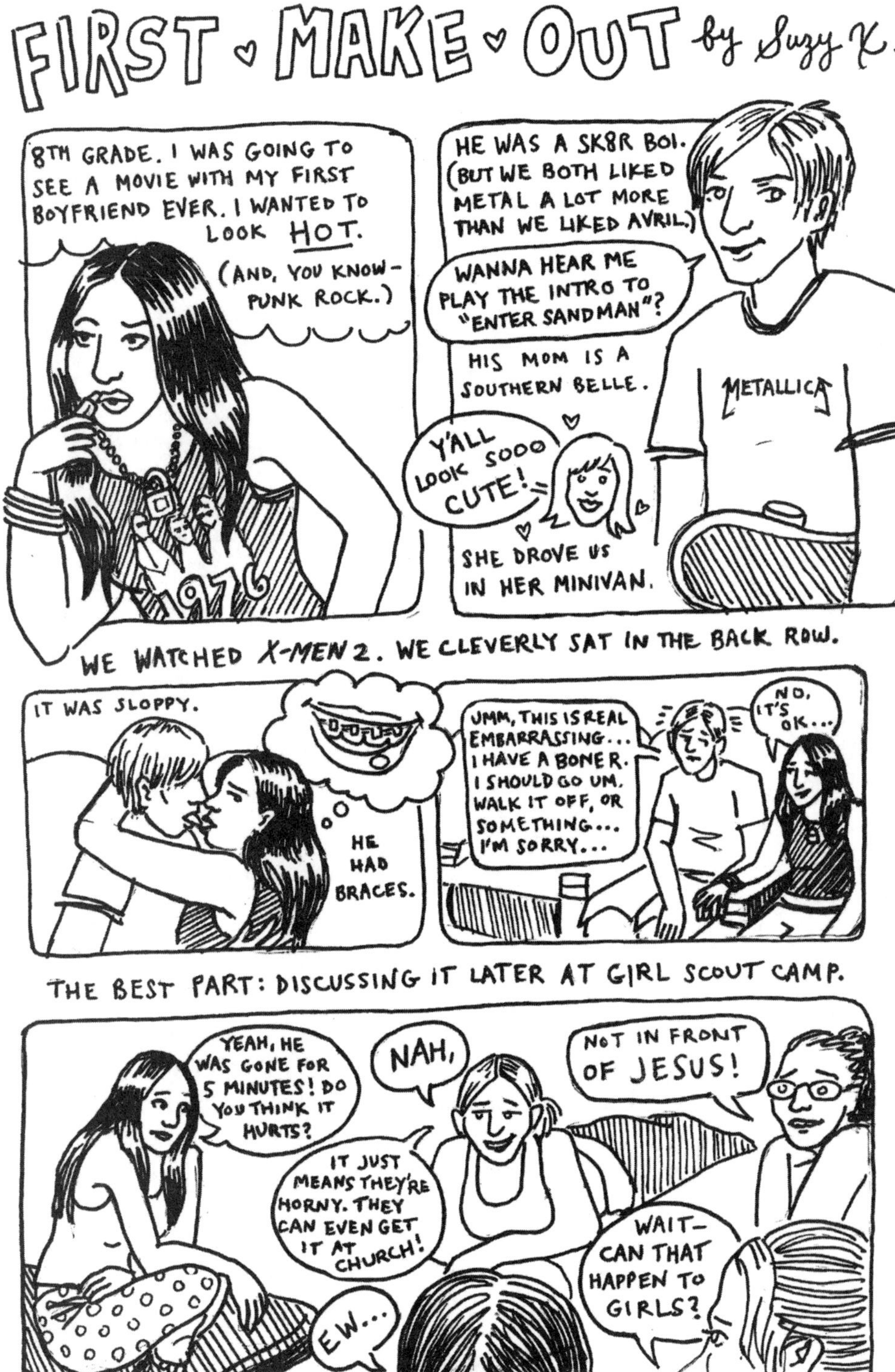
FIRST ♡ MAKE ♡ OUT by Suzy K.
8TH GRADE. I WAS GOING TO SEE A MOVIE WITH MY FIRST BOYFRIEND EVER. I WANTED TO LOOK HOT.
(AND, YOU KNOW- PUNK ROCK.)
1976
HE WAS A SK8R BOI. (BUT WE BOTH LIKED METAL A LOT MORE THAN WE LIKED AVRIL.)
WANNA HEAR ME PLAY THE INTRO TO "ENTER SANDMAN"?
METALLICA
HIS MOM IS A SOUTHERN BELLE.
Y'ALL LOOK SOOO CUTE!
SHE DROVE US IN HER MINIVAN.
WE WATCHED X-MEN 2. WE CLEVERLY SAT IN THE BACK ROW.
IT WAS SLOPPY.
HE HAD BRACES.
UMM, THIS IS REAL EMBARRASSING... I HAVE A BONER. I SHOULD GO UM, WALK IT OFF, OR SOMETHING... I'M SORRY...
NO, IT'S OK...
THE BEST PART: DISCUSSING IT LATER AT GIRL SCOUT CAMP.
YEAH, HE WAS GONE FOR 5 MINUTES! DO YOU THINK IT HURTS?
NAH,
IT JUST MEANS THEY'RE HORNY. THEY CAN EVEN GET IT AT CHURCH!
NOT IN FRONT OF JESUS!
WAIT- CAN THAT HAPPEN TO GIRLS?
EW...

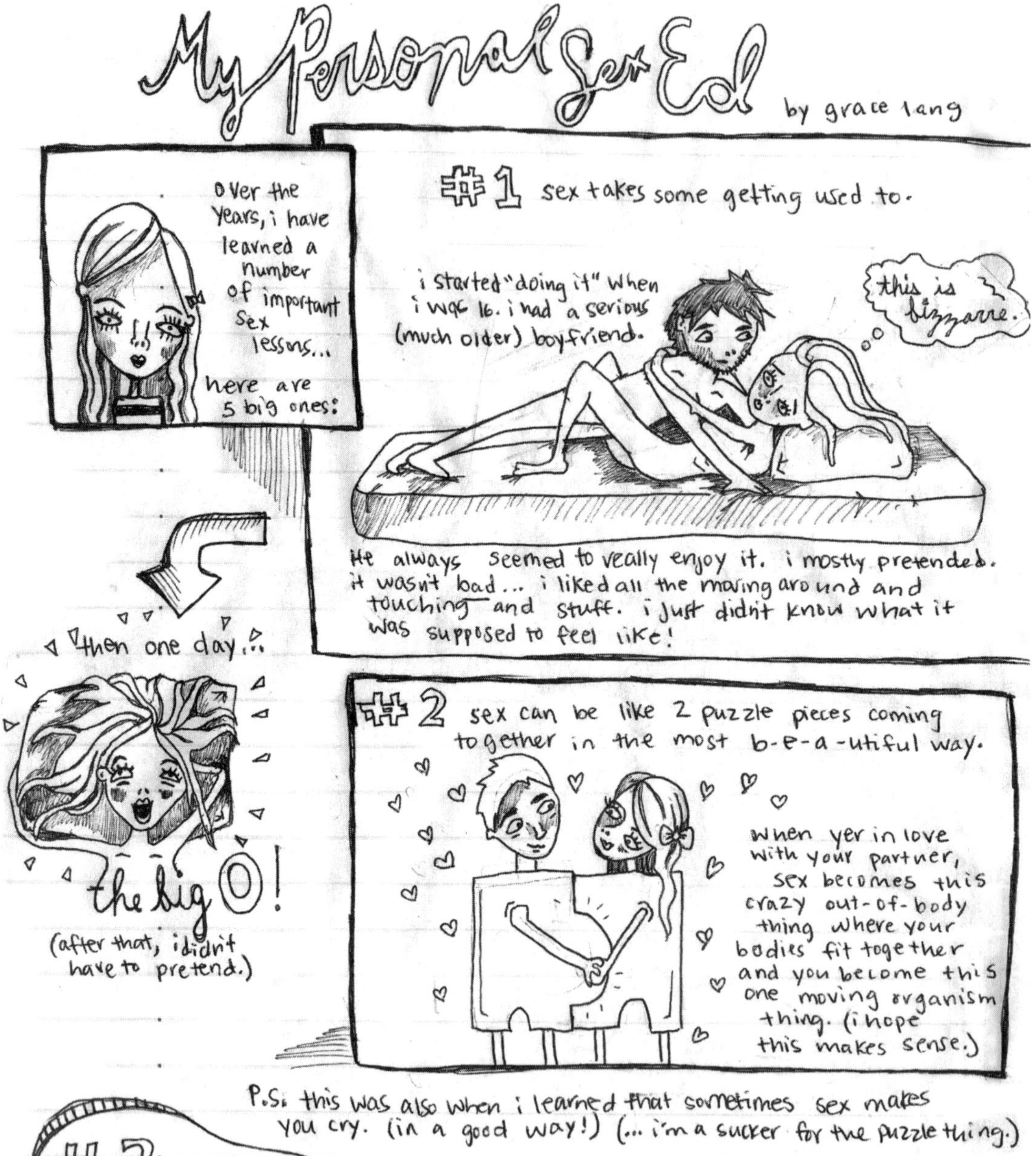

My Personal Sex Ed
by grace lang

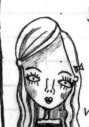

Over the years, i have learned a number of important sex lessons...

here are 5 big ones:

#1 sex takes some getting used to.

i started "doing it" when i was 16. i had a serious (much older) boyfriend.

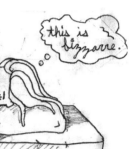

this is bizzarre.

He always seemed to really enjoy it. i mostly pretended. it wasn't bad... i liked all the moving around and touching and stuff. i just didn't know what it was supposed to feel like!

then one day...

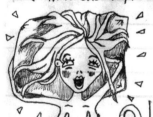

the big O!

(after that, i didn't have to pretend.)

#2 sex can be like 2 puzzle pieces coming together in the most b-e-a-utiful way.

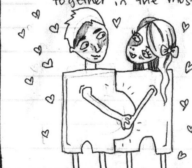

when yer in love with your partner, sex becomes this crazy out-of-body thing where your bodies fit together and you become this one moving organism thing. (i hope this makes sense.)

P.S. this was also when i learned that sometimes sex makes you cry. (in a good way!) (... i'm a sucker for the puzzle thing.)

#3 games/fantasies are normal. AND FUN!

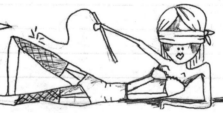

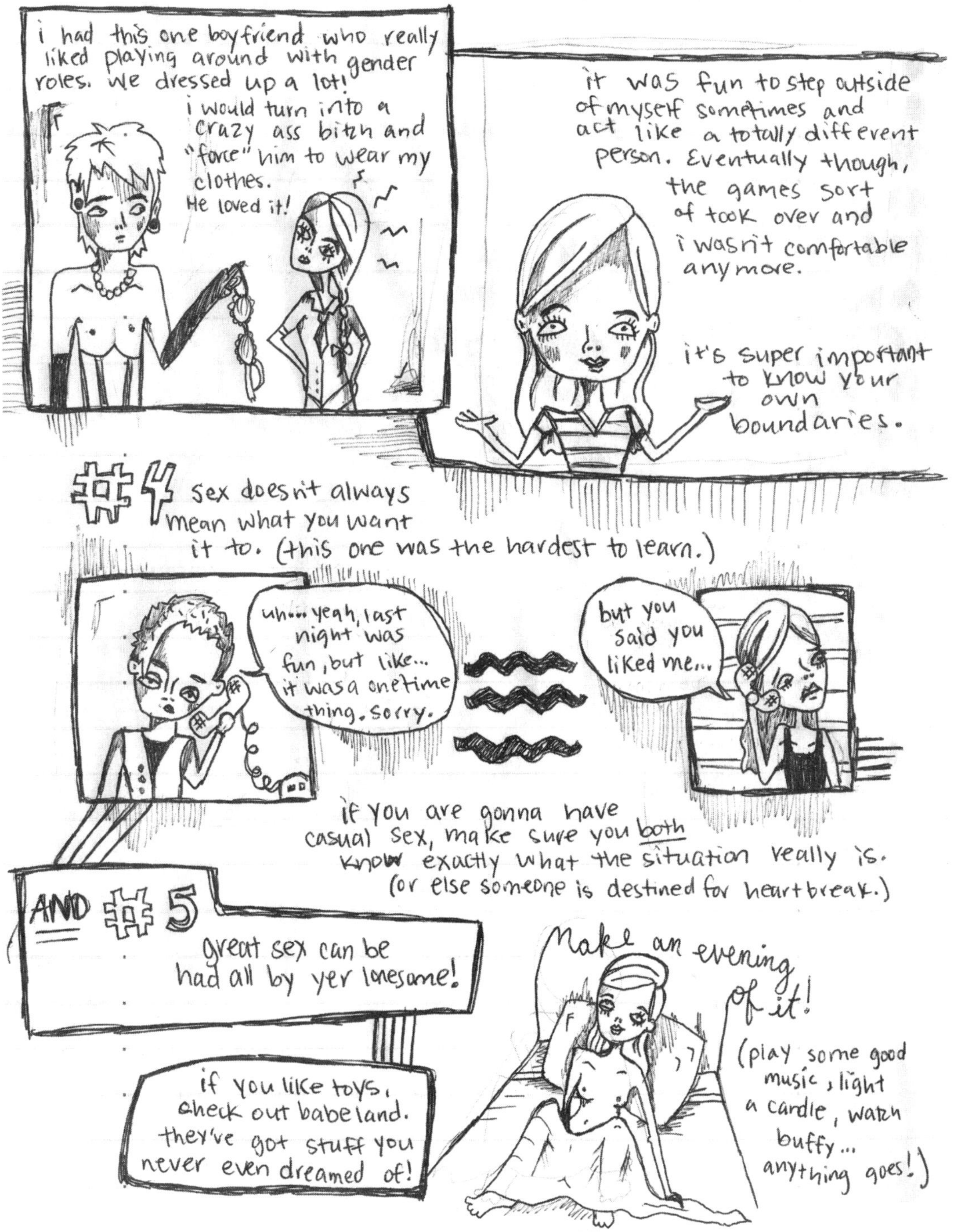

i had this one boyfriend who really liked playing around with gender roles. we dressed up a lot!
i would turn into a crazy ass bitch and "force" him to wear my clothes.
He loved it!
it was fun to step outside of myself sometimes and act like a totally different person. Eventually though, the games sort of took over and i wasn't comfortable anymore.
it's super important to know your own boundaries.
#4 sex doesn't always mean what you want it to. (this one was the hardest to learn.)
uh... yeah, last night was fun, but like... it was a one time thing. sorry.
but you said you liked me...
if you are gonna have casual sex, make sure you both know exactly what the situation really is. (or else someone is destined for heartbreak.)
AND #5
great sex can be had all by yer lonesome!
Make an evening of it!
if you like toys, check out babeland. they've got stuff you never even dreamed of!
(play some good music, light a candle, watch buffy... anything goes!)

CHAPTER TWO:

BODIES

SAIYA

She loosens her tie and pulls it quickly through her collar. I look straight into her eyes just before she wraps it around my head, blindfolding me. She had a long night at work, and she is still working quickly, pulling my hands together and fastening my wrists with her belt. I can feel the breeze coming through the window, hear the muffled music from the neighbor's television, all the noise on the street, but it's quiet in the room except for my breath quickening. I can hear her work shirt hit the floor, and I grin when I hear her trip getting out of her jeans. "Hey, give me a break!" she says, kissing me once, slowly. Then she moves around me and pulls me down to the bed. I cannot tell how long we wrestle until the sun starts rising, the sky changing its clothes from navy to denim to sweatpants blue.

She's not really my type. That is what I like about her. I would not have known, in passing, that she was someone I would like to roll around with. At first I was unsure of her; I did not know how to read her. When we started talking, though, I felt it, the pull. I felt completely drawn to her. Around her I became funnier, more charming, my hair shining brighter, and my laugh more musical. I liked who I was with her. She made me feel like butter on hot toast.

She surprised me the first time we slept together. She was bossy, really bossy, and it was fun. I could whine and pout and she would just keep bossing me around. She was the driver. I found myself relaxed and relieved. Since I felt that we were

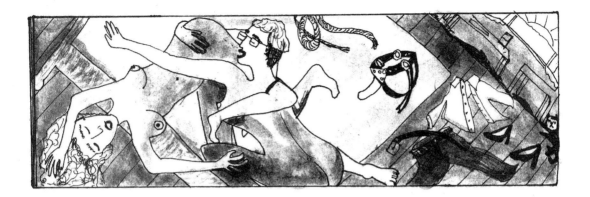

evenly matched, there was an immediate trust between us. It felt completely safe. This made room to play around.

She changed the way I felt about my body. Mine was drawn to hers. In the beginning I judged her too soon as an unlikely person for me to be with. In fact, she was very important to me. She set me free because she was commanding and yet sweet, impulsive yet considerate, powerful yet soft. There was still a lot of uncertainty hiding in my limbs. They reached out in question, and she just grabbed them and took hold.

LIZA

For all my sexual misadventures, there were also some great experiences. In junior high, I visited an old friend, Twyla, who lived in California. Unlike mine, her friends were doing a lot of drugs and also having a lot of sex. On this particular evening, we were hanging out in some boy's living room and the group was exchanging gossip that I knew nothing about. A boy who was a head shorter than all the girls started bragging about the great sex he was having. Even though I hadn't been talking before, I fell even more silent. This was the first time I had heard girls and boys talk about sex, together. I sank deep into the sofa.

Twyla laughed at him and said, "That's not what I heard. Riley told me that every time you guys do it, she has to masturbate after you leave."

There was a blanket on my lap and I pulled it up to my chin and tried to pretend I was asleep. I struggled to keep my eyes closed.

"She masturbates?" the boy asked.

All the girls in the room laughed. Twyla answered, "Of course."

"Do you all masturbate, too?" he asked, even more astonished.

I think I might have started sweating. Back home, my friends never talked about sex, because we weren't having any, or masturbation, because it was supposed to be gross. My friend Twyla and the rest of the girls took turns talking about the different ways they masturbated. One girl's favorite tool was a spoon. A *spoon*. For a month, I would remember this girl every time I ate soup.

And then I heard about the bathtub faucet. Apparently, this girl wedged her ass up against the end of the bathtub and pressed her feet on the edge at either side of the faucet. Water flowed out, hitting her clitoris until she orgasmed. I still had the blanket around me, but I no longer pretended to be asleep. This was the most exciting story I had ever heard. I wanted to go home and try it, immediately.

A week and a half later, my parents finally left the house for an extended period of time. I locked the bathroom door and started the shower. I followed my normal routine, but instead of turning off the water when I was finished, I pushed the knob so the water came out of the bottom faucet instead. I sat down and stretched out. Hot water flowed over my toes. Slowly, I inched my butt closer to the end of the tub, toward the water. I reclined and leaned on my forearms. My butt slapped against the porcelain wall, pushing my vulva up. The water hit my clit. It was too much and I jumped back for a second, but then slipped back into position. I slowly started to rock back and forth. It took about two minutes of water pressure for my muscles to contract and I felt the internal vibrations of my first orgasm.

SAIYA

The Atlas bone and the Eustachian tube are both named after mythical old white guys, and yet we all have to carry them around in each of our bodies. Anatomical terms are constantly evolving and changing to suit the demands of modern medicine. Why shouldn't we be able to name parts of our own bodies to suit ourselves?

Mythical and comic book characters have an easier time with this. They have extra limbs, impossibly enormous hair and lashes, wings, and whatever else they need to get through the day. They are drawn outrageously, drawn into their everyday drag, and don't need to explain it. They have always been good role models, strutting down the page in an ambitious outfit. If a bodysuit is so tight it looks painted on, that is the uniform they were given. If they are blue, it's understood.

The first time I went home with a trans man, I was really nervous. I felt like if I did something wrong while we were together, I would never live it down. I had recently been to a workshop about using better consent, so I wanted to ask everything out loud. I realized halfway through the encounter that this urge was butting heads with the question of what language to use during sex. My attempts at good consent that night all trailed off, as if they were being sucked down a wind tunnel—"Do you want me too . . ." "Would it feel good if . . ." "How are you feeling when . . ."—until he looked me straight in the eye and said, "It's a COCK."

I blushed and nodded. I wished I had just known what to say without being told what he preferred and how to name it. But then I realized that what I should have done right away was just ask. It wasn't my choice anyway; it was his. It made me think about the importance of choosing for yourself how to talk about your body. I realized I hated certain words that were thrown at me all the time, but that I had gotten used to: *nice boobs, so pretty, curvy, princess, nice rack, hey red, does the carpet match the curtains?* Like someone with a bullhorn trying to sneak their way under my clothes and give a guided tour.

Nature cannot be used as an argument for or against alternative modes of sexuality, because we are living in a wide new civilization where artificial insemination, egg donation, and surrogate mothering can make even heterosexual family planning a scientifically advanced endeavor. The decision to augment one's own body can be related to gender, but more generally, it is about presentation, how a body presents itself to the world.

I wish I had been taught about all the possibilities as a kid, all the interesting stories of queer lovers and caretakers, whether they were making babies in test tubes or cuddling like swans. I had to seek them out.

DURING THIS EARLY EXPLORATION with different people and different kinds of sex, I unearthed three new memories. I was curious about them, wondering why they surfaced when they did, because I felt that I was doing really well. They came back suddenly, as if from a long trip, huffing loudly and dropping their bags. They are all from a long time ago, but stayed hidden until recently. They came back during sex: the first when someone put a hand on my hip in a certain way, the second when someone pulled my hair a little too hard, the third when someone put both of his hands on my neck.

It was almost Christmas, and my sister and I had gone into the city to visit a friend of hers. The cold was bitter, and the edges of our scarves were pulled up to meet the edges of our hats, leaving only a small melon wedge–shape for our eyes. The apartment was too hot and too dry, so we peeled down to our T-shirts and joined the dance party in the living room. At one point I took a break and looked out the window, gazing far down below at the antlike people walking their antlike dogs. An older guy whom I had seen around once or twice came up next to me, and I instinctually moved away a little. He said something obvious about how high up we were. I fake-smiled and walked into the kitchen, pretending to need a glass of water. The night rolled on, and everyone finally found some sort of corner to curl up in and sleep. My sister was down the hallway in a different room. I lay down on a foldout couch in the corner next to the Christmas tree and fell asleep immediately.

I woke up and it was that time just before sunrise. My throat was dry and the room was quiet, but I could feel that someone on the bed next to me was also awake. I felt stiff and stayed in the exact same position, trying to pretend that I was still sleeping. Then I felt a hand on my hip. It rested there and then moved up under my shirt. Without changing position, with my arms crossed over my chest, I simply rolled off the bed, like a mummy falling out of a sarcophagus. The room was silent and I lay there until the gray morning, my hair tangled in the low branches of the Christmas tree, looking at my fishbowl reflection in a shiny red ornament.

The next memory was silent and badly lit. I was dancing in a different living room. There was barely any furniture. A stupid guy was there; I knew him from the park where we hung out. He was annoying, touching my hair and pulling it like a little kid. He pulled me into a room with another girl. He pulled off his shirt and pulled ours off, too. The other girl left the room, laughing. The memory faded out after that: all I remembered was the crack of light under the door and the dull beat of the music from the other room.

The third was from a fight I had with my first boyfriend. The sun was rising and we were sitting on my bed. He was in pain, crying, and I was anguished and trying to make him stop. He put my hand on his throat and told me to choke him. I didn't want to, but it seemed like the only thing he wanted me to do. I pressed my hand into his throat until he was gasping for breath, and he reached over and took my neck into both of his hands, pressing down until I felt my vision going watery and dizzy. I thrashed and gasped and he let go.

I think I pressed these memories down for a while because they were so unsettling, so nauseating. Each time, I had no control over the way I was being touched. Each time, something went too far. I can feel each vividly, because it is connected to a part of my body. All I have to do is visit them: when someone touches my hip or pulls my hair or puts a hand on my neck. Sometimes it feels silly, that these are the places that are the most sensitive. But memories live in the body.

LIZA

I have faked orgasms with almost all of my partners since my earliest sexual experiences. I faked it before I knew what an orgasm felt like, though I learned early on that the pressure of the water flowing out of the bathtub faucet did more for me than a penis, finger, or tongue ever could. Somehow my sexual partners are less accepting of this, especially men.

Most of my relationships last only a night. Some of the men I have been with don't even attempt to bring me to climax. This may be because of inexperience, nervousness, apathy, or liquor. Whatever the reason, they're not invited back. However, there are more generous lovers, and I appreciate their effort and passion.

After we engage in various types of sex, I can sense they're waiting for my body to do something about their continued effort. If I tell these one-night lovers that I'm not going to cum, many take it as a challenge. They ignore my preexisting knowledge of my body and believe they have the magic fingers and tongues needed. The only thing worse than a partner's determination is the unbearable pressure to let my body go.

One time, I told this guy I was not going to orgasm. It was three o'clock in the morning and he was high on cocaine. "Well, I'm not going to stop till I make you cum," he said, as if he were a knight on a white horse, come to rescue me from my frigid self. I looked at his big bristly face. A few faked gasps and muscle contractions seemed like my only option.

It feels worse when I'm exploring my sexual limits with someone I care deeply about. I want my body to explode simply from their touch.

"Does that feel good?"

"Yes. Yes, almost there. Wait. Stop. I think I just have to pee. Sorry. Sorry."

There is so much pressure to make your bodies share that special moment. They want it. I want it. Sometimes, it is just easier to fake it.

MUFFIN TOP
BACK FAT
WRINKLY
HAIR
FLAB
SCARS
SHORT
SMELL
ZIT
I FORGET THAT MY BODY NEEDS TO BE LOVED, NOT CRITICIZED.
MASTURBATION IS ONE WAY TO SHOW MY BODY LOVE!
LOVE YOUR SELF
THERE IS NO WRONG WAY TO MASTURBATE, SO JUST PLAY AROUND.

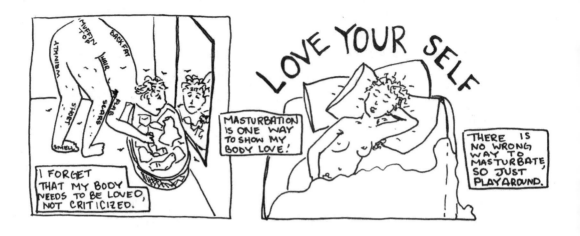

Once, I was casually having sex with a friend of mine. Each time we went to bed together he asked how he could make me orgasm. Every time I had to tell him that it probably wasn't going to happen, but I still enjoyed being fingered and receiving head. He liked to watch me masturbate. Even though I told him, multiple times, that I wasn't going to have an orgasm, he was still always waiting for me to cum. I cared for this person and I felt ashamed that despite his valiant effort, my body was not going to do what we wanted it to do. So I inevitably faked an orgasm. Then I felt guilty. He often was unable to maintain an erection. So, most nights, neither of us would cum. I still regret not being honest with him, because even without orgasms, our sex was really wonderful. It was a long engagement of tender touching mixed with rough play. We would spoon all night in the winters. In the summer, when New York apartments are hotter and more humid than outside, we lay naked on opposite sides of the bed, feet entwined. In the mornings we got coffee and went our separate ways.

In my early twenties, I became a lot more confident during sexual interactions. If I brought someone home to my room, I would ask if it was okay if I used my vibrator to cum. One time a woman asked if I had another toy she could use. I did, but it was a battery-operated vibrator and I had no way of sanitizing it that night. She said that was fine because we could just put a condom over it. We masturbated each other and then ourselves and I orgasmed several times. She left before the sun came up. My experience with her was fleeting but extremely important to my future sex life. Afterward, I never felt uncomfortable asking a partner if we could introduce a new element into our lovemaking.

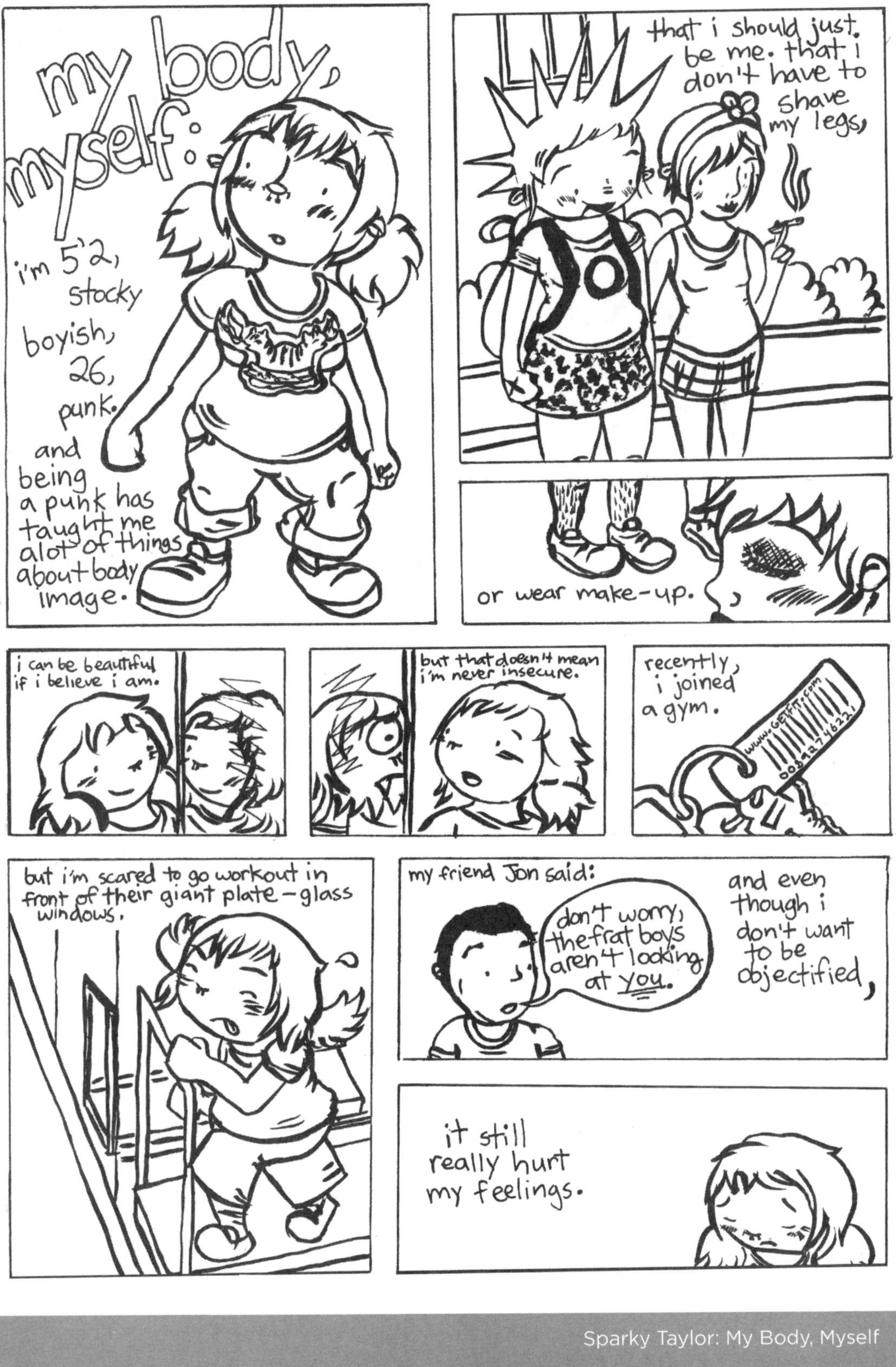

my body, myself:
i'm 5'2, stocky boyish, 26, punk.
and being a punk has taught me alot of things about body image.
that i should just be me. that i don't have to shave my legs,
or wear make-up.
i can be beautiful if i believe i am.
but that doesn't mean i'm never insecure.
recently, i joined a gym.
www.GETFIT.com
but i'm scared to go workout in front of their giant plate-glass windows.
my friend Jon said:
don't worry, the frat boys aren't looking at you.
and even though i don't want to be objectified,
it still really hurt my feelings.

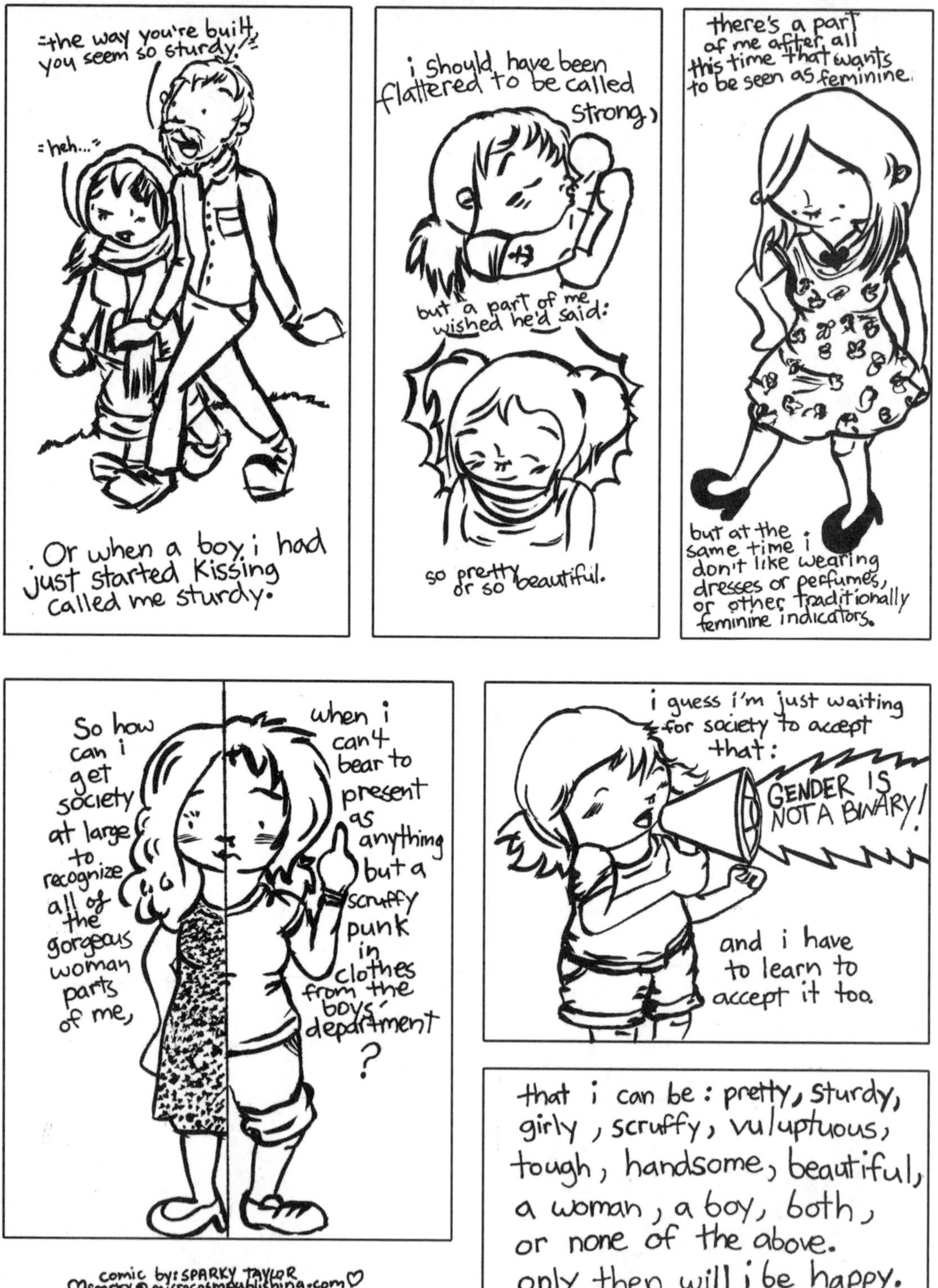
= the way you're built, you seem so sturdy! =
= heh... =
Or when a boy i had just started Kissing called me sturdy.
i should have been flattered to be called strong,
but a part of me wished he'd said:
so pretty or so beautiful.
there's a part of me after all this time that wants to be seen as feminine.
but at the same time i don't like wearing dresses or perfumes, or other traditionally feminine indicators.
So how can i get society at large to recognize all of the gorgeous woman parts of me,
when i can't bear to present as anything but a scruffy punk in clothes from the boys' department?
i guess i'm just waiting for society to accept that:
GENDER IS NOT A BINARY!
and i have to learn to accept it too.
that i can be: pretty, sturdy, girly, scruffy, vuluptuous, tough, handsome, beautiful, a woman, a boy, both, or none of the above. only then will i be happy.
comic by: SPARKY TAYLOR
sparky@microcosmpublishing.com

i've always had trouble with my

BODY

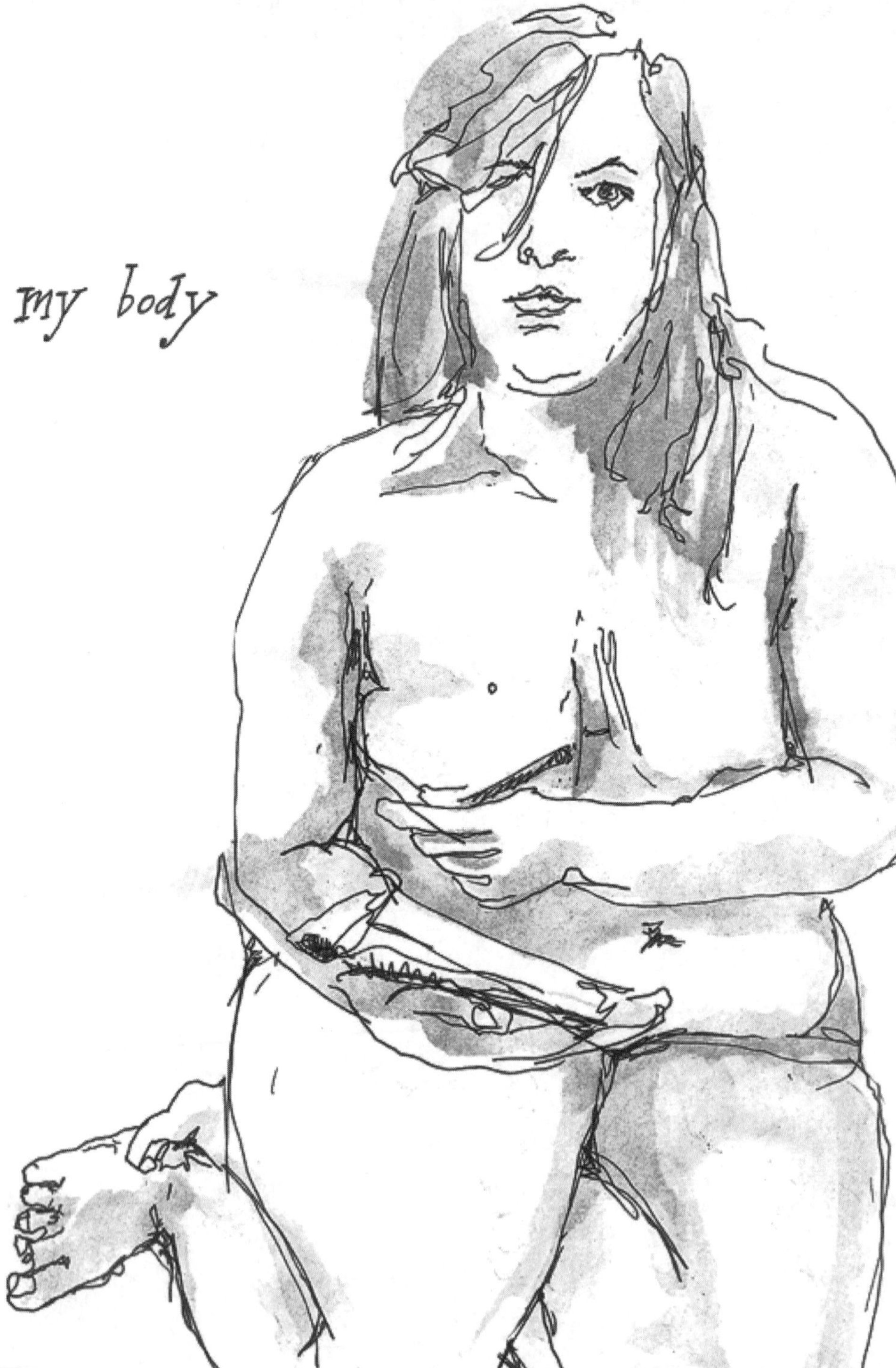
my body

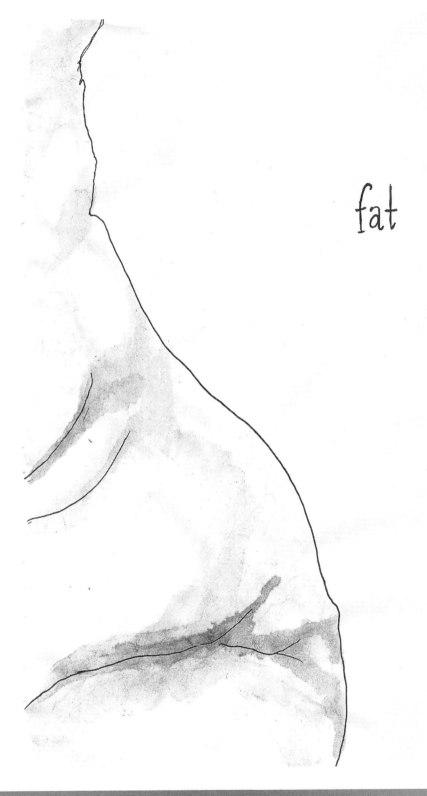

fat

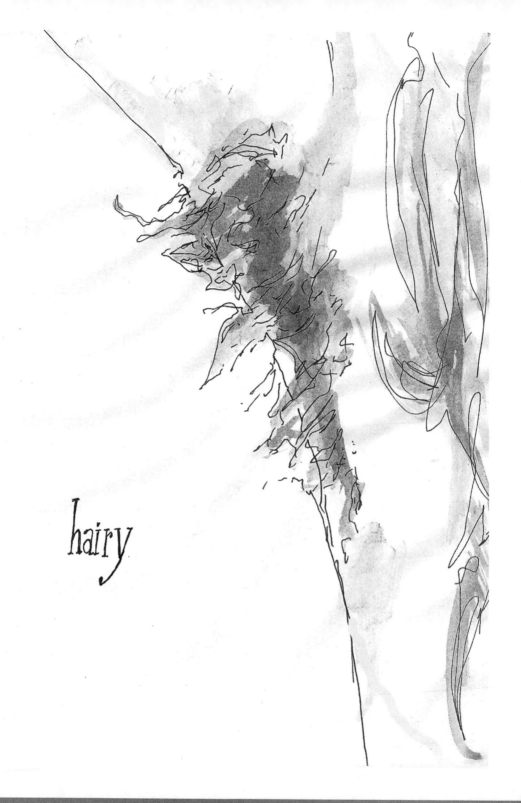

hairy

things get complicated for me when other bodies get involved...

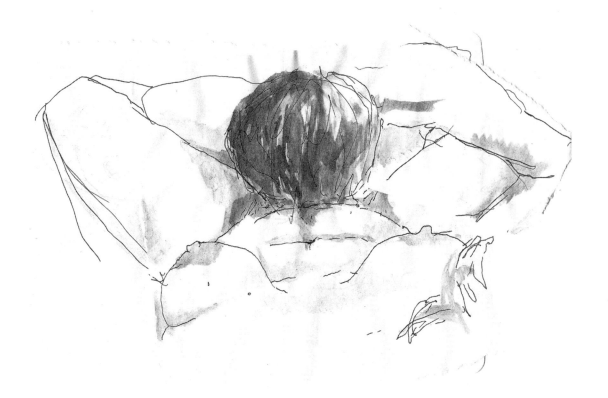

when a body tells you you're beautiful

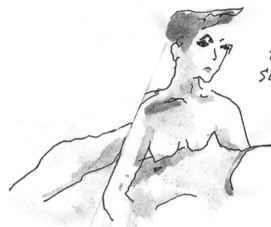

then a body tells you there is something wrong with you

when you can't do what that body wants your body to do.

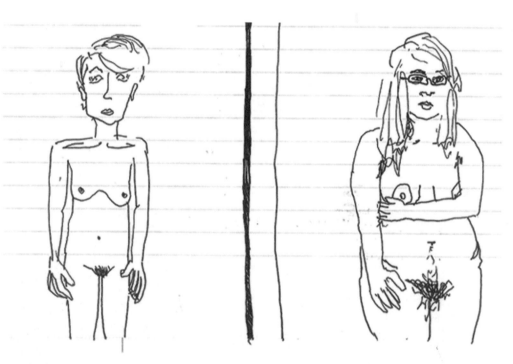

things get even more complicated when the other body is no longer involved.

So i've never had an orgasm.

i spent so long resenting my body -- talking shit about it, trying to change it -- it's no wonder it doesn't feel like giving.

i'm 23 yrs old.
i've never had an orgasm.
I'm learning to love my body.
it will all work out.

Kate. 2010.

Holes.
by cynthia ann schemmer
home base
the bible
my first serious sexual relationship spawned the realization that our society lacks decent sex ed. a huge factor in this personal story is that my first boyfriend was raised as a born again christian. this influenced a lot of our sexual relations,
ONE HOLE?
HA HA HA!
So, imagine my reaction when he revealed to me that females only have ONE HOLE to perform our many bodily functions!!!
Just think about having to pee out of our vaginas...
A FOREVER FLOW OF PISS.

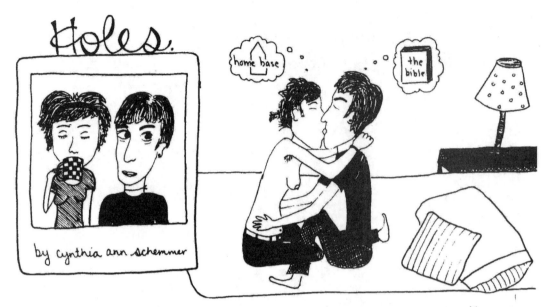

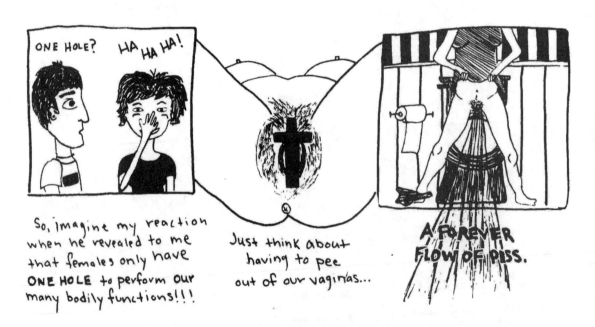

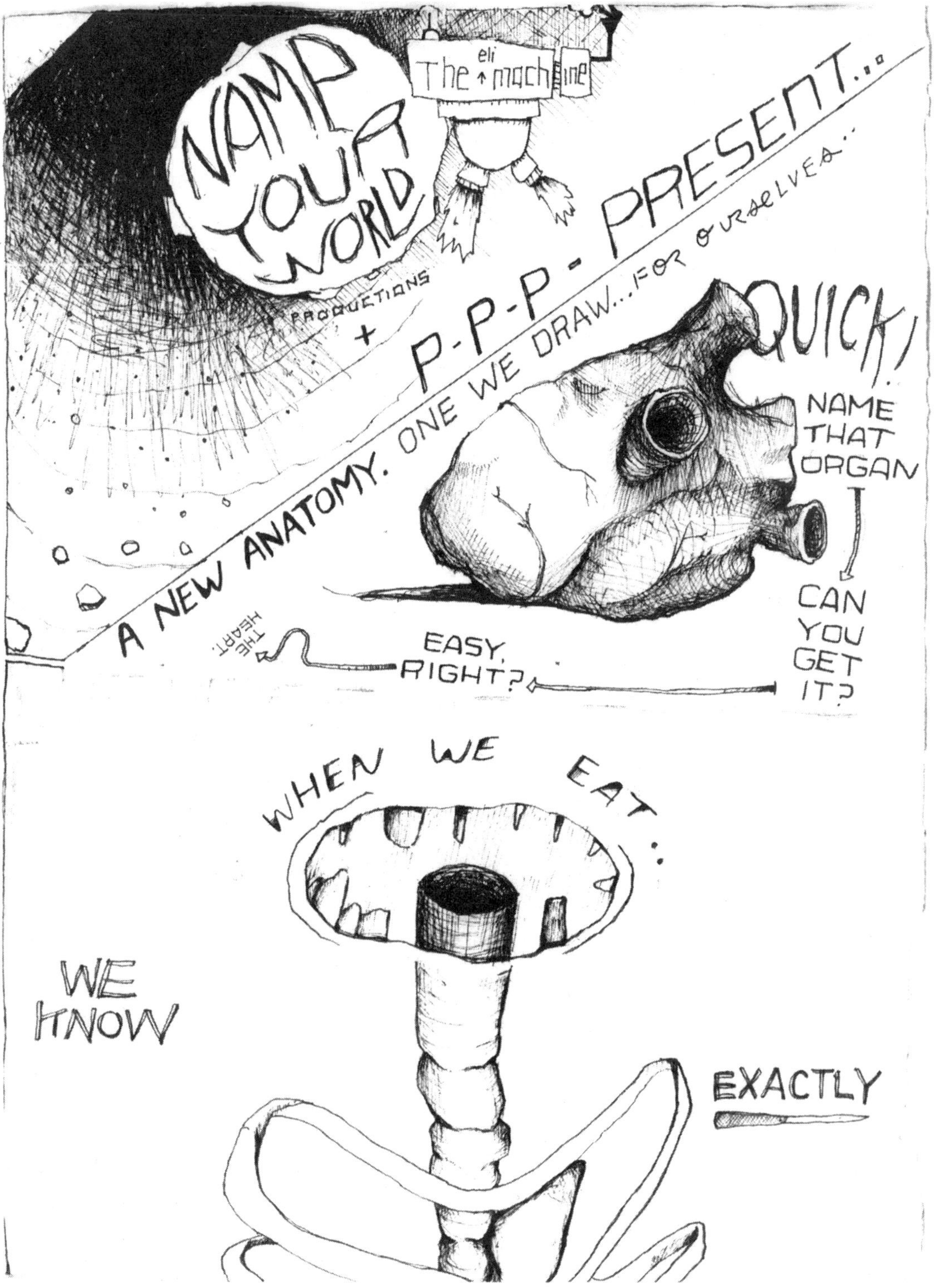
NAME YOUR WORLD
The eli machine
PRODUCTIONS
+
P-P-P - PRESENT..
A NEW ANATOMY. ONE WE DRAW... FOR OURSELVES..
QUICK!
NAME THAT ORGAN
CAN YOU GET IT?
EASY, RIGHT?
THE HEART.
WHEN WE EAT..
WE KNOW
EXACTLY

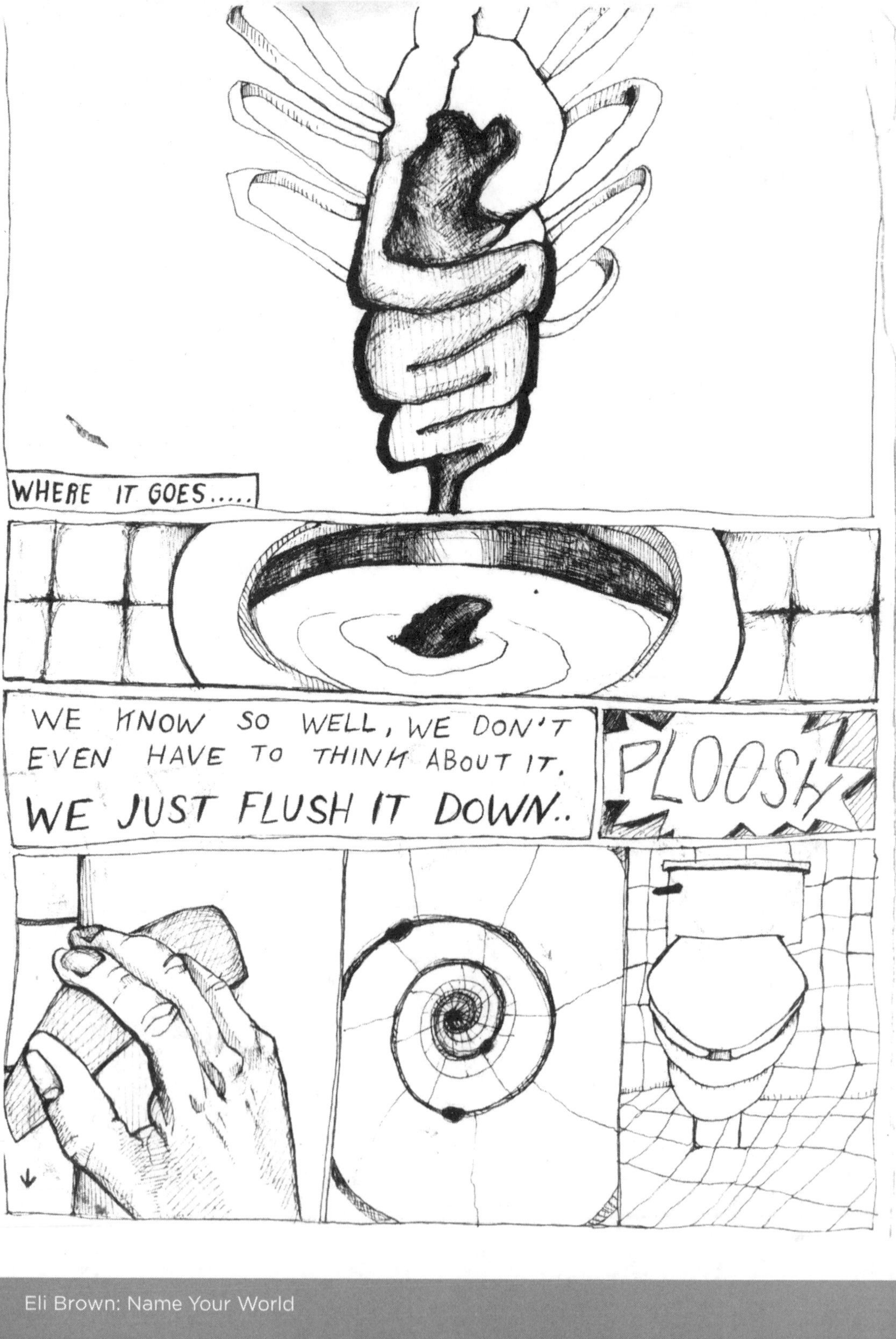
WHERE IT GOES.....
WE KNOW SO WELL, WE DON'T EVEN HAVE TO THINK ABOUT IT.
WE JUST FLUSH IT DOWN..
PLOOSH

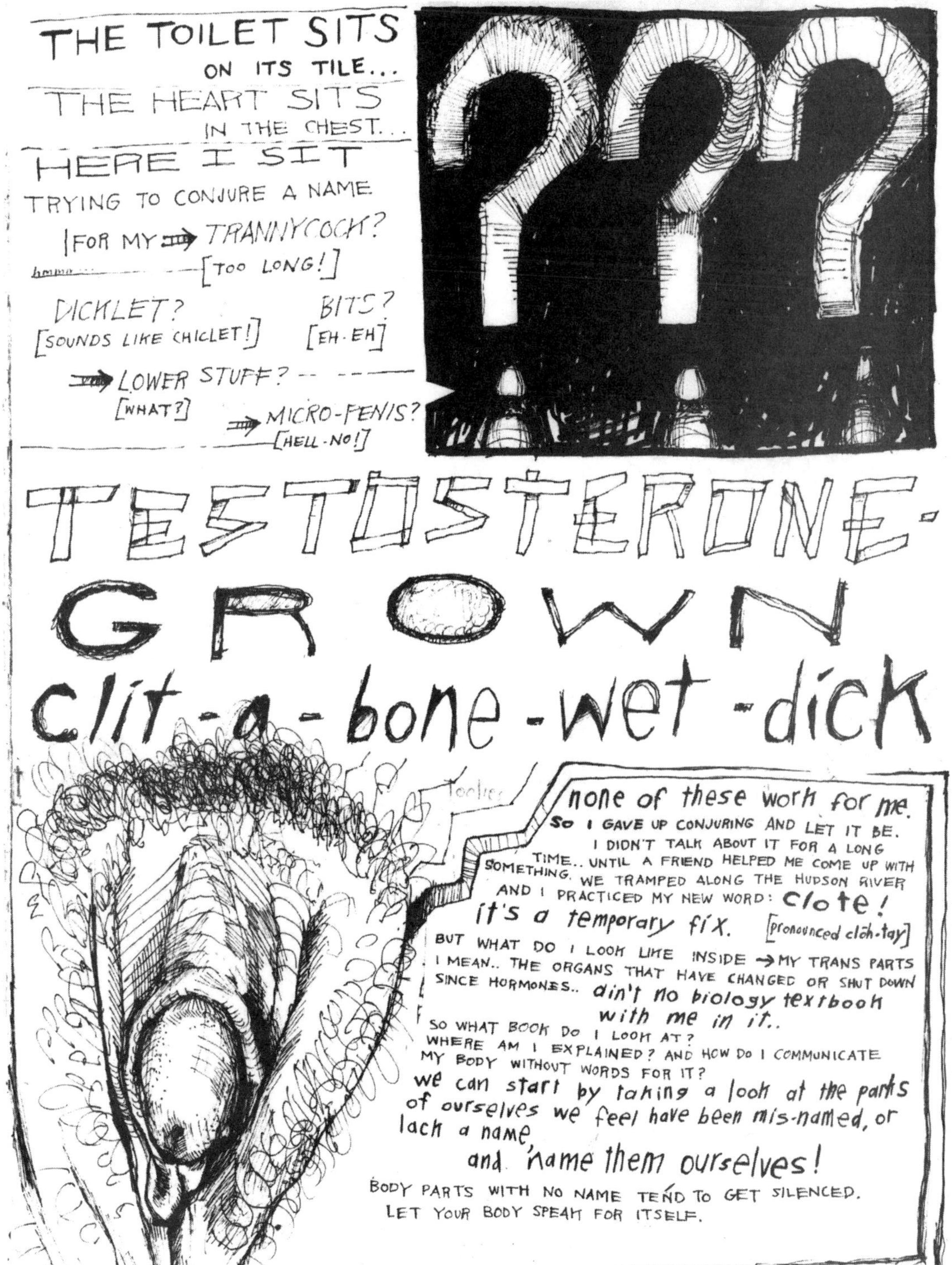
THE TOILET SITS
ON ITS TILE...
THE HEART SITS
IN THE CHEST...
HERE I SIT
TRYING TO CONJURE A NAME
FOR MY → TRANNYCOCK?
hmmm... [TOO LONG!]
DICKLET? [SOUNDS LIKE CHICLET!]
BITS? [EH-EH]
→ LOWER STUFF? [WHAT?]
→ MICRO-PENIS? [HELL-NO!]
???
TESTOSTERONE-
GROWN
clit-a-bone-wet-dick
none of these work for me.
SO I GAVE UP CONJURING AND LET IT BE. I DIDN'T TALK ABOUT IT FOR A LONG TIME.. UNTIL A FRIEND HELPED ME COME UP WITH SOMETHING. WE TRAMPED ALONG THE HUDSON RIVER AND I PRACTICED MY NEW WORD: clote!
it's a temporary fix. [pronounced clōh-tay]
BUT WHAT DO I LOOK LIKE INSIDE → MY TRANS PARTS I MEAN.. THE ORGANS THAT HAVE CHANGED OR SHUT DOWN SINCE HORMONES.. ain't no biology textbook with me in it..
SO WHAT BOOK DO I LOOK AT? WHERE AM I EXPLAINED? AND HOW DO I COMMUNICATE MY BODY WITHOUT WORDS FOR IT?
we can start by taking a look at the parts of ourselves we feel have been mis-named, or lack a name, and name them ourselves!
BODY PARTS WITH NO NAME TEND TO GET SILENCED.
LET YOUR BODY SPEAK FOR ITSELF.

MY SMALL boobs

As a fat kid, I was born with boobs

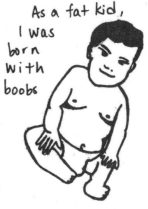

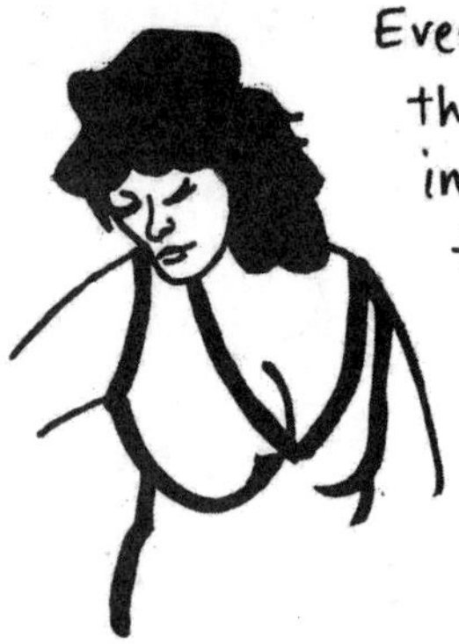

Everyone thought that I would grow into them and take after my mother.

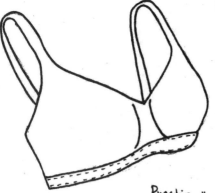

In middle school they were the same size as they had been since I was two years old.

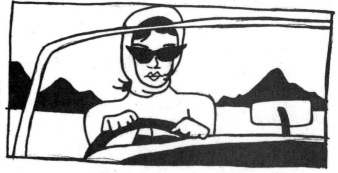

I didn't think I'd be an adult until I got breasts (and learned how to drive)

I tried push-up padded bras with disastrous results. Not even a AA fit and I had an awkward space between the padding and my chest.

... Practically cavernous.

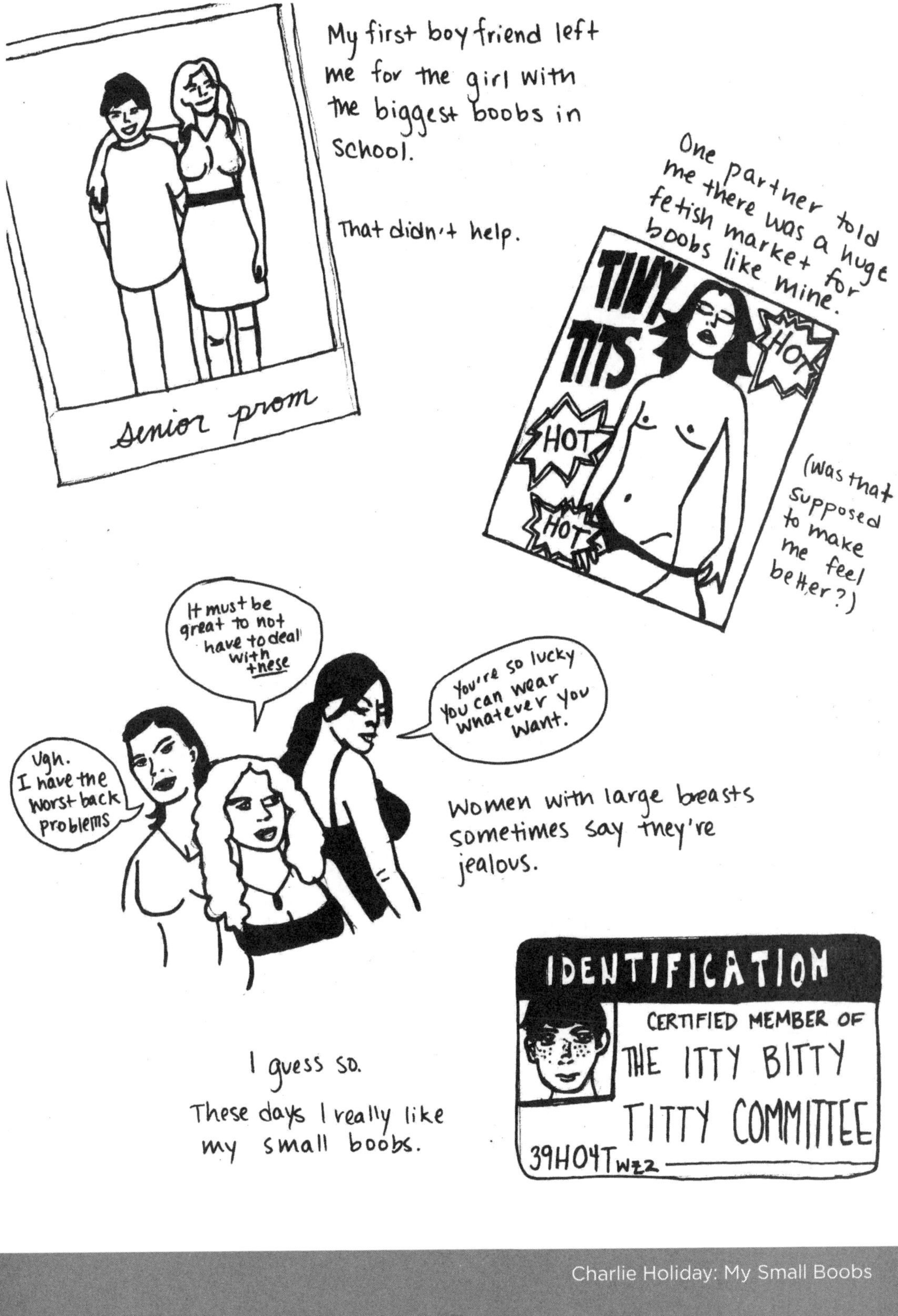
My first boyfriend left me for the girl with the biggest boobs in school.
That didn't help.
senior prom
One partner told me there was a huge fetish market for boobs like mine.
TINY TITS
HOT
HOT
HOT
(was that supposed to make me feel better?)
Ugh. I have the worst back problems
It must be great to not have to deal with these
You're so lucky you can wear whatever you want.
Women with large breasts sometimes say they're jealous.
I guess so.
These days I really like my small boobs.
IDENTIFICATION
CERTIFIED MEMBER OF
THE ITTY BITTY TITTY COMMITTEE
39H04Twz2

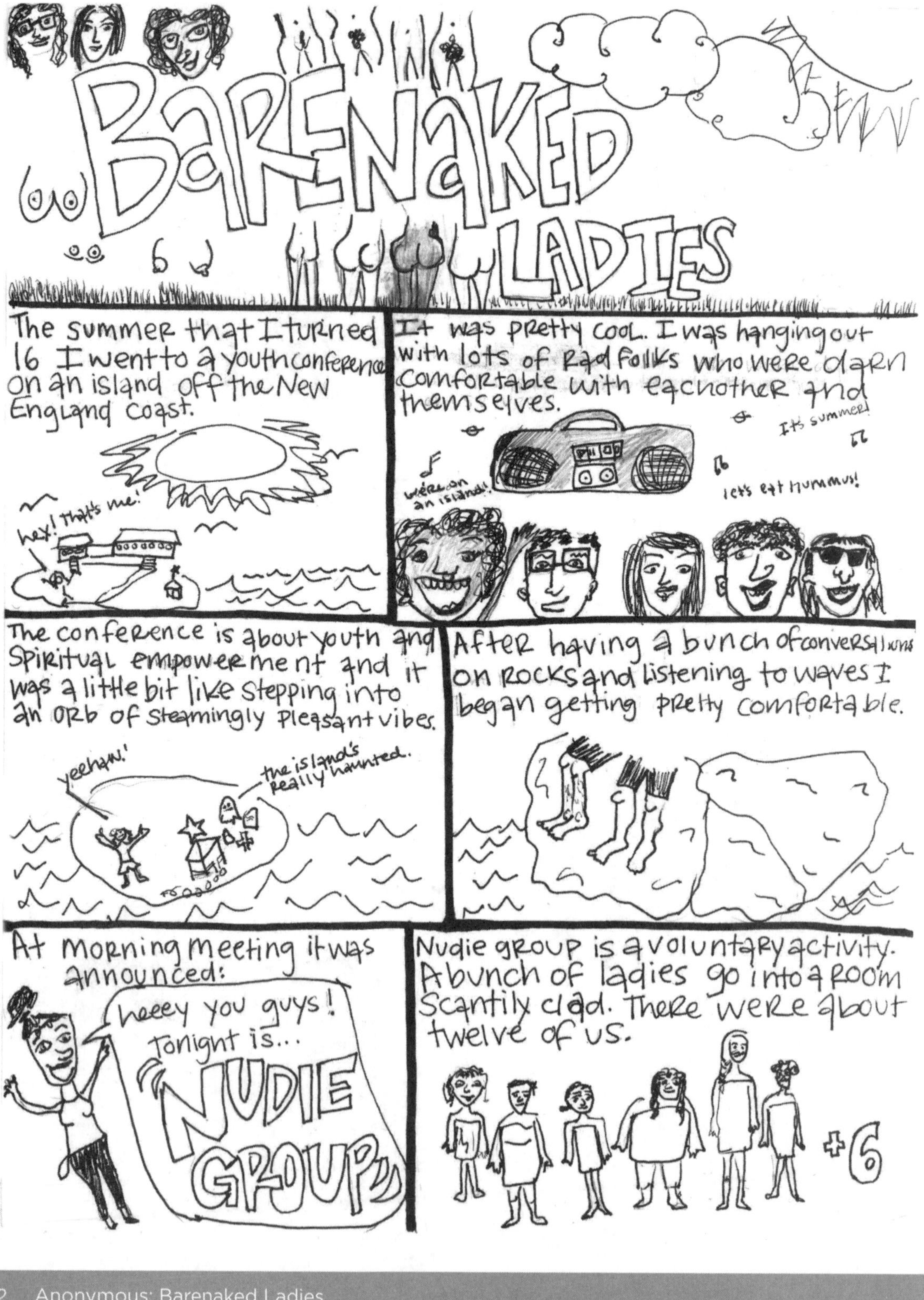
BARENAKED LADIES
The summer that I turned 16 I went to a youth conference on an island off the New England coast.
hey! that's me!
It was pretty cool. I was hanging out with lots of Rad folks who were darn comfortable with eachother and themselves.
It's summer!
we're on an island!
let's eat hummus!
The conference is about youth and Spiritual empowerment and it was a little bit like stepping into an orb of steamingly pleasant vibes.
yeehaw!
the island's really haunted.
After having a bunch of conversations on rocks and listening to waves I began getting pretty comfortable.
At morning meeting it was announced:
heeey you guys! Tonight is... NUDIE GROUP
Nudie group is a voluntary activity. A bunch of ladies go into a room Scantily clad. There were about twelve of us.
+6

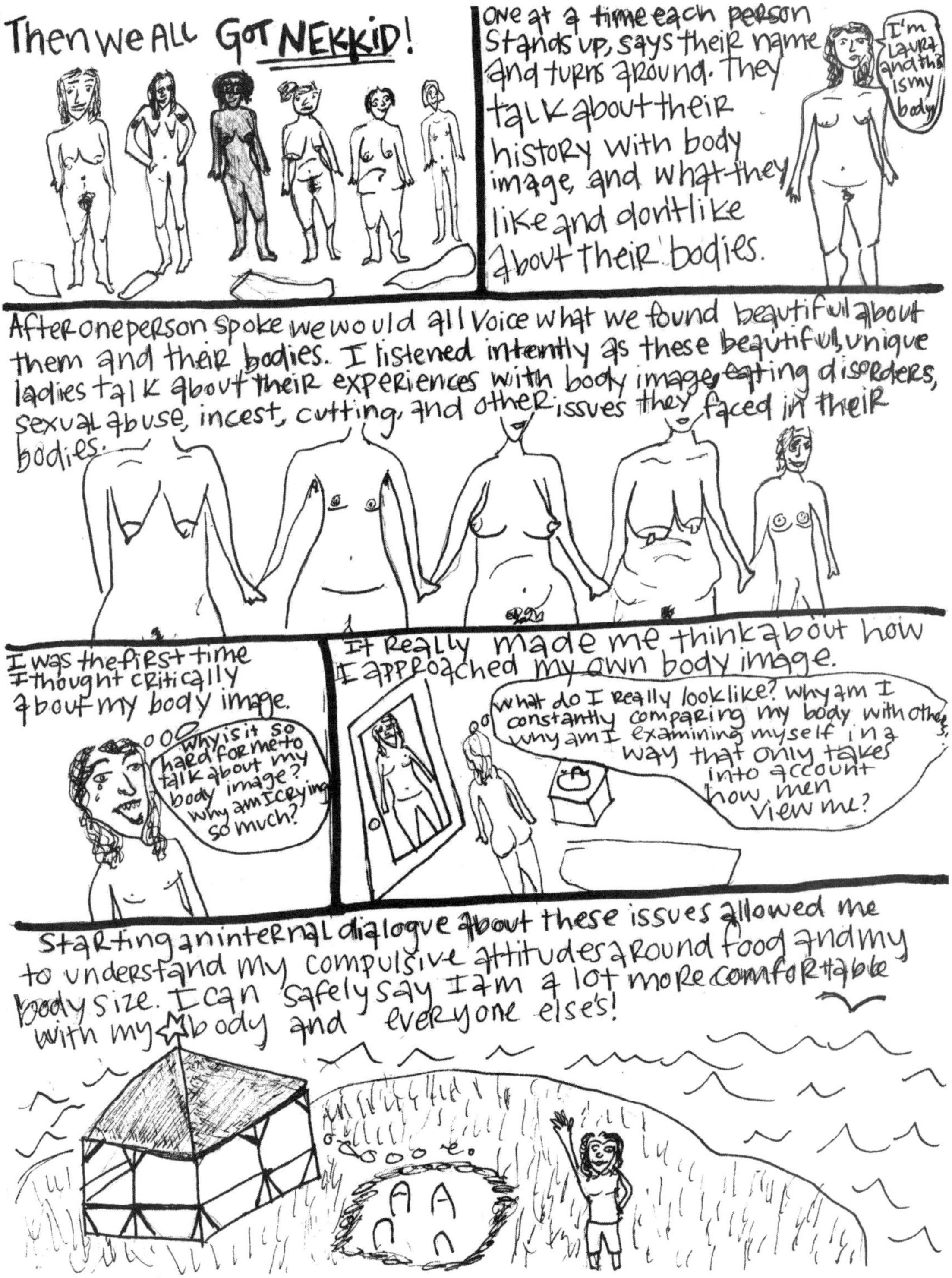
Then we ALL GOT NEKKID!
One at a time each person stands up, says their name and turns around. They talk about their history with body image, and what they like and don't like about their bodies.
I'm Laura and this is my body
After one person spoke we would all voice what we found beautiful about them and their bodies. I listened intently as these beautiful, unique ladies talk about their experiences with body image, eating disorders, sexual abuse, incest, cutting, and other issues they faced in their bodies.
I was the first time I thought critically about my body image.
Why is it so hard for me to talk about my body image? Why am I crying so much?
It really made me think about how I approached my own body image.
What do I really look like? Why am I constantly comparing my body with others? Why am I examining myself in a way that only takes into account how men view me?
Starting an internal dialogue about these issues allowed me to understand my compulsive attitudes around food and my body size. I can safely say I am a lot more comfortable with my body and everyone else's!

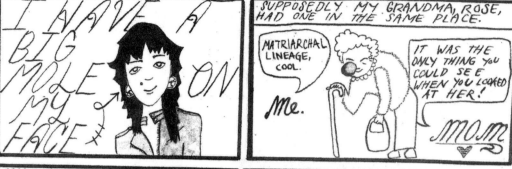

MOLE

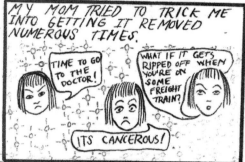

I HAVE A BIG MOLE ON MY FACE ↗

SUPPOSEDLY MY GRANDMA, ROSE, HAD ONE IN THE SAME PLACE.

MATRIARCHAL LINEAGE, COOL.

Me.

IT WAS THE ONLY THING YOU COULD SEE WHEN YOU LOOKED AT HER!

MOM ♥

MY MOM TRIED TO TRICK ME INTO GETTING IT REMOVED NUMEROUS TIMES.

TIME TO GO TO THE DOCTOR!

WHAT IF IT GETS RIPPED OFF WHEN YOU'RE ON SOME FREIGHT TRAIN?

ITS CANCEROUS!

SHE SCARED ME OF IT.

DON'T TOUCH IT! IT'LL GET BIGGER!

I USED TO STARE AT IT IN THE MIRROR UNTIL IT WAS THE ONLY THING I COULD SEE AND I WOULD REGRET NOT GETTING IT REMOVED

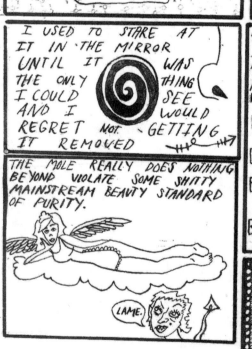

THE MOLE REALLY DOES NOTHING BEYOND VIOLATE SOME SHITTY MAINSTREAM BEAUTY STANDARD OF PURITY.

LAME.

IT STILL SOMETIMES CONFUSES ME WHY I HAVENT. I ALREADY HAVE TONS OF MARKS FROM OTHER DECISIONS...

☑ shitty tattoo — moon-sister

☑ cheep fake tooth

☑ drunken bike wreck facial scarr

☑ scars from popping zits

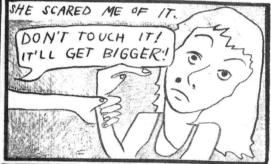

BUT THEN, EVERYONE CAN CHOOSE PART OF THEIR BODY TO FREAK-OUT ABOUT...

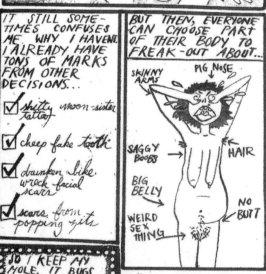

SKINNY ARMS

PIG NOSE

SAGGY BOOBS

HAIR

BIG BELLY

WEIRD SEX THING

NO BUTT

SO I KEEP MY MOLE. IT BUGS MY MOM, GROSSES OUT DOUCHIE DUDE-BRAHS, GIVES ME A MEMORABLE FACE... I'M "THE GIRL WITH THE MOLE" & I THINK ITS PUNK AS FUCK.
YOURS TRULY,
SARAH ROSE

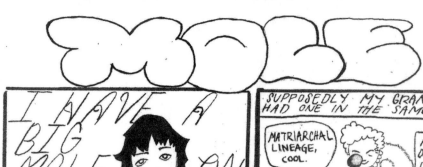

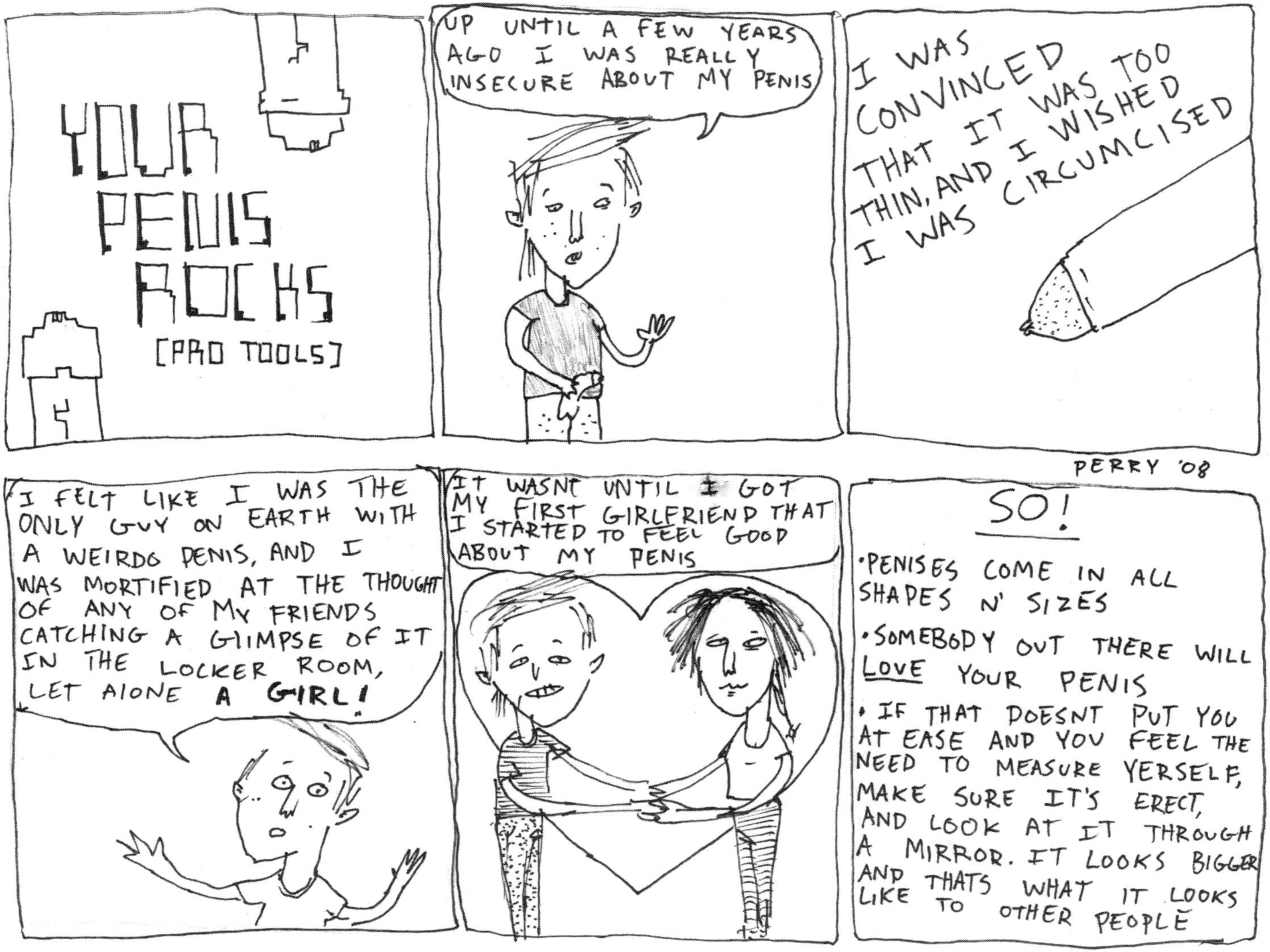
YOUR PENIS ROCKS
[PRO TOOLS]
UP UNTIL A FEW YEARS AGO I WAS REALLY INSECURE ABOUT MY PENIS
I WAS CONVINCED THAT IT WAS TOO THIN, AND I WISHED I WAS CIRCUMCISED
PERRY '08
I FELT LIKE I WAS THE ONLY GUY ON EARTH WITH A WEIRDO PENIS, AND I WAS MORTIFIED AT THE THOUGHT OF ANY OF MY FRIENDS CATCHING A GLIMPSE OF IT IN THE LOCKER ROOM, LET ALONE A GIRL!
IT WASNT UNTIL I GOT MY FIRST GIRLFRIEND THAT I STARTED TO FEEL GOOD ABOUT MY PENIS
SO!
•PENISES COME IN ALL SHAPES N' SIZES
•SOMEBODY OUT THERE WILL LOVE YOUR PENIS
•IF THAT DOESNT PUT YOU AT EASE AND YOU FEEL THE NEED TO MEASURE YERSELF, MAKE SURE IT'S ERECT, AND LOOK AT IT THROUGH A MIRROR. IT LOOKS BIGGER AND THATS WHAT IT LOOKS LIKE TO OTHER PEOPLE

SOMATIC MEMORIES: BODY TRIGGERS

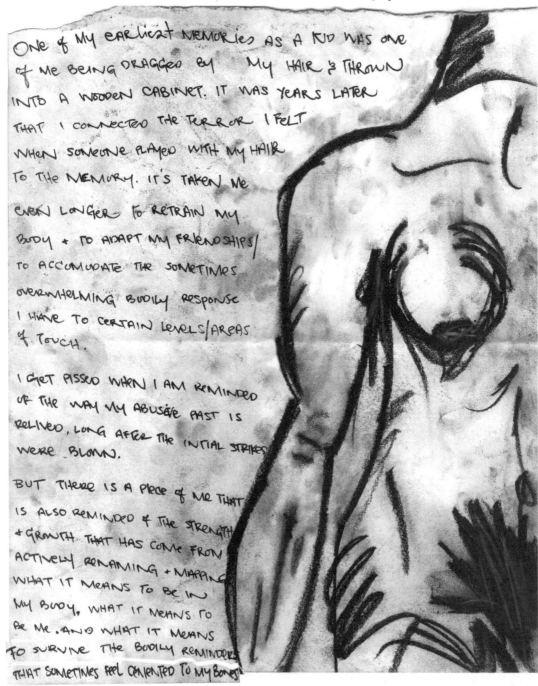

ONE OF MY EARLIEST MEMORIES AS A KID WAS ONE OF ME BEING DRAGGED BY MY HAIR & THROWN INTO A WOODEN CABINET. IT WAS YEARS LATER THAT I CONNECTED THE TERROR I FELT WHEN SOMEONE PLAYED WITH MY HAIR TO THE MEMORY. IT'S TAKEN ME EVEN LONGER TO RETRAIN MY BODY & TO ADAPT MY FRIENDSHIPS/ TO ACCOMODATE THE SOMETIMES OVERWHELMING BODILY RESPONSE I HAVE TO CERTAIN LEVELS/AREAS OF TOUCH.

I GET PISSED WHEN I AM REMINDED OF THE WAY MY ABUSIVE PAST IS RELIVED, LONG AFTER THE INITIAL STRIKES WERE BLOWN.

BUT THERE IS A PIECE OF ME THAT IS ALSO REMINDED OF THE STRENGTH & GROWTH THAT HAS COME FROM ACTIVELY RENAMING + MAPPING WHAT IT MEANS TO BE IN MY BODY, WHAT IT MEANS TO BE ME. AND WHAT IT MEANS TO SURVIVE THE BODILY REMINDERS THAT SOMETIMES FEEL CEMENTED TO MY BONES.

CHAPTER THREE:

HEALTH

SAIYA

In ninth grade I was required to take a class on public speaking and speech writing. This class, which was taught by the coldest woman I had ever known, slowly devolved into a perilous game of what felt like Russian roulette. There was one day a week when we made speeches one by one at the front of the class, and you never knew who might be the one to break down in the middle of a speech. There was always at least one person who did. These days filled my stomach with dizzying fear. I could see it mirrored in the eyes of my classmates at the front of the room, especially the girls. Their small voices shook and their hands clenched the edges of their essays or scratched pointlessly at the hips of their jeans. Rachel Rominsky actually fainted during one of her speeches, falling sideways onto the linoleum. I had never seen anyone faint before. It was the only thing the rest of the class could remember about her speech. I was petrified and took it as a bad omen. My problem was that every time I tried to make a speech, I started to cry. It did not matter what my speech was about. I would get up to make my argument for gun control or to describe how to build a toy rocket and my face would fill with hot rage that welled up and then overflowed. It was as if the whole class was summoning the tears, waiting patiently for me to melt. I could feel an impending crisis coming over the horizon. I had to find a way out, and the only way to get out of making speeches was to get a note from a therapist.

The therapist talked slightly, too slowly, like how it sounded when I nudged the record player down just a millimeter, not far enough to distort the voice into sludge. Her lipstick was a luminescent pink, throwing the rest of the room into a colorless drought in the winter light coming through the bay window behind me. I thought about those old black-and-white photographs where only one part is tinted with color.

She did not seem interested in the speech class or why I had made an appointment. Instead she asked, with a slight narrowing of the eyes, "How do you usually feel?" I could feel her looking at me, too hard. It was a lot like the audience of the class. I could feel the tears welling up. "Sad," I said, "just sad."

"All the time?" she demanded.

"Kind of, yeah." I felt shamed. Sad, what a dumb thing to be. My sadness was compounded by the murky mystery of why I was sad in the first place.

She kept asking other things, more and more, things that had nothing to do with making speeches. I began to wonder why I was there at all. I wanted to get out as quickly as possible. I felt exposed.

She pushed on, asking about my parents, my little brother and big sister, and also about how I felt about my body, the changes in my body, and boys at school.

This was too much. I felt anger rise in my throat like puke. It was none of her business, the crazy stuff going on in my body. Boys at school were hardly a threat compared to the girls, who both obsessed and terrified me. I might have wanted to talk about all of that stuff, but I felt like a mouse that had been cornered. It wasn't safe there; I was being judged. She was a doctor but she was also a stranger whom I had come to for help. She was pushing beyond what I had come to talk about. I had not given her permission to mine my psyche.

"I'm just sad, OK?"

She pursed her lips together, making the pink disappear for a moment. She scribbled for a little while in her notebook and then ripped the note out and handed it to me. I knew I had disappointed her. I had not given her any meat, any gristle.

LIZA

My clothes were in a pile in a corner of the room. I was dressed in a thin robe, but already the robe and the sheet they gave me had bunched around my waist. My feet were up above my body in the stirrups. I was in that uncomfortable bared position, at the doctor's office, for the loop electrosurgical excision procedure, or LEEP.

LIZA, I WENT TO THE GYNO AND SHE GAVE ME TWO SPECULUMS
UM... HOW DOES THIS WORK?
WE SAW OUR CERVIXES
IF DOCTORS SEE YOUR CERVIX...
SHOULDN'T YOU TAKE A PEEK?

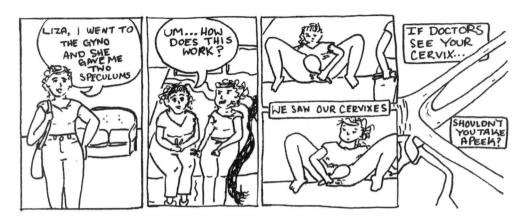

My heart was working fast, not because of the stress but because of the epinephrine the nurse had shot directly into my cervix. The sting rippled across my muscles and up my body. Epinephrine is adrenalin, which was why it quickened my heart and I couldn't find my breath. It also helps control bleeding. I tensed and inched up on the table, away from the edge. One woman pushed me back down so the other could open my legs wider. I got chills from her cold hands, even through the plastic gloves. They injected me with a couple more substances to numb the pain.

They pressed a sticky electrosurgical dispersive pad on my exposed thigh. The pad had a wire coming out of it. This device grounded my body, so I wouldn't be electrocuted from the inside of my vagina. Then they went to work.

It didn't hurt. I felt the warmth but not the pain. The doctor used electricity to slice the surface of my cervix with a wire loop. She pulled three pebble-sized chunks of flesh out of me. Each chunk of my cervix was stored in a clean, clear receptacle and labeled. The solution in the containers quickly turned dark red as my cervix bled. Eyes wide, I was still unable to find my breath.

"We've got it all. Please make a follow-up appointment in four weeks and don't put anything in your vagina."

Blood entered and exited my heart just as quickly as during the procedure. It would take an hour for the epinephrine to expire. My mother drove me away from the hospital to my grandmother's home. I leaked a spicy yellow.

At home, I was brewing coffee in my lower back. The pulsing of my blood had finally slowed and with it the adrenaline and anesthesia. I began to feel the residual burn, like menstrual cramps. My movement was limited. I was afraid that sneezing would be detrimental because of the muscle spasm it caused. Of course, I craved a hot water bottle heater and chocolate.

After two days, I finally discharged the grounds of the coffee I had brewed on the first day. I pulled a clump of dried blood that lived in a mucus sack out of my vagina. Those grounds crawled out for a few more days. I bled for weeks, slowly. It took me six months to feel comfortable putting anything up my vaginal canal, even my fingers.

Two months before the loop electrosurgical excision procedure, I was in the same doctor's office for a cervical biopsy. That was when they told me I was HPV-positive. The nurse said, "You don't have to inform past partners about your status. HPV is the STI to have. The majority of sexually active women have it. You're young; it will probably go away."

Four weeks before the biopsy, that same HPV had caused a high-grade squamous intraepithelial lesion on my cervix that led to an abnormal Pap smear that led to the biopsy. The biopsy did not solve the persistent dysplasia, but it did indicate the need for the electrosurgical procedure. My pre-cancer was cut, carved, torn, and burned out of me successfully, but the procedures and products of the HPV lingered.

SAIYA

It started when I was seventeen years old. Any time I was really stressed out or especially dirty, or sometimes right before my period, I would have my own personal version of hell right there in my own crotch. It just plain hurt. I did not know what was going on at all, so I prepared for the worst, too embarrassed and scared to actually get myself checked out.

This went on for over six months, and I was at the end of my rope. Plus, I made the fatal mistake of looking up my symptoms online, something one should never do since many symptoms are the same for both mild and severe conditions, it seems. I figured I probably had herpes or some other lifelong condition for which there was no cure. I figured my short sex life was over, replaying the greatest hits in my mind. I thought longingly of the upholstered couch where I had last played in the garden of innocent ignorance. I knew that all I needed to do was get some professional help, but I held myself back for a long time. I feared a replay of past visits to professionals and the distinct feeling of being judged.

Finally, I went to get tested for STIs and had a full physical examination at a clinic. This took a great deal of courage. I realized, though, that only a medical professional with more knowledge of the body than I had would be able to take a look and decide my true fate.

The physician said that all I had was a recurrent yeast infection, a common problem. "Don't worry, hon," she reassured me. Her name was Janice, and to me she was a savior, with a tattoo of a fairy on her ankle and long, bleached hair braided down her back.

Still, I had a lot of questions and a lot to learn about what was actually going on. I knew yeast was in foods I liked and that I might have to eat less of them. "But . . . I love spaghetti," I groaned to myself, picturing little microbial beasts taking over my body one by one. Yeast was everywhere, and I would have to learn to keep it in balance. I learned to take notice of the early warning signs of an infection. Someone would call to invite me to a party and I would force myself to tell them, "I would normally say yes, but I am feeling a little run down." I also started eating lots of fermented foods, which contain probiotics and help regulate the internal environment. I still have a lot to learn about how my body works and what is right for me, but I've come a long way.

Looking back, I see that the malady itself was not what did me in: it was my inability to face up to the problem and deal with it. I let it go on and on because I was scared. I was paralyzed by embarrassment.

The last place I will ever have sex.
YOU'RE GONNA DIE!!!

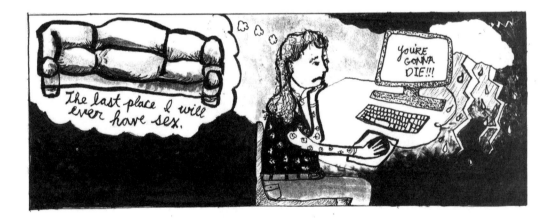

LIZA

To not share my positive HPV status and my experiences with my past partners and the women in my life would be a choice to add to the silence. Not all women with HPV have the same experience. Many must undergo more hospital visits, more painful procedures, and more serious health repercussions. Even more do not have access to early screening, medical procedures, or close familial support because of a litany of political and social systems, including enforced structural racism and classism. I did not want to contribute to the already high risk that my partners and my partners' partners were facing.

My positive HPV status was one of two opportunities I've had to make those uncomfortable phone calls to past sexual partners. Years before my HPV, I also tested positive for trichomoniasis, which is treated with antibiotics. While these calls were embarrassing and sometimes hurtful, I've never regretted making them. It is an opportunity to take something we're forced to feel vulnerable and shameful for and turn it into a proud experience. Being sexually active, often while drunk, with multiple partners for over a decade means, yes, STIs are just going to be part of the package. We need destigmatization, honest conversations, and a discourse of shamelessness.

SAIYA

Healthy living is complex. The cereal commercials say that all you need to do is stay true to a breakfast brand and jog around a field with your dog. The brochures in the doctor's office tell you how to put on a condom or recognize an STI.

To really be healthy, though, you must also pay attention to what is happening in your mind. How you think and feel affects your body.

When I was most depressed, I was also the weakest physically that I have ever been. I had strep throat three times and mononucleosis, and was on the verge of dropping out of high school. My sickly body and my troubled mind were slow-dancing.

Since then, I have had to totally reinvent ways to stay healthy. I learned that if I start feeling beaten down I have to put on the brakes, start drinking tea, and go to sleep early. My antidote to feeling sick is taking it easy, and my antidote to feeling down is being around friends, being social. But if I feel anxious or depressed, it is difficult to take it easy because doing so means secluding myself from my friends and receding into my head. With feelings of physical sickness and mental strife often going hand in hand for me, it is a tenuous balance. My health depends on a task: to find comfort in being by myself, to find the joy in slowing down.

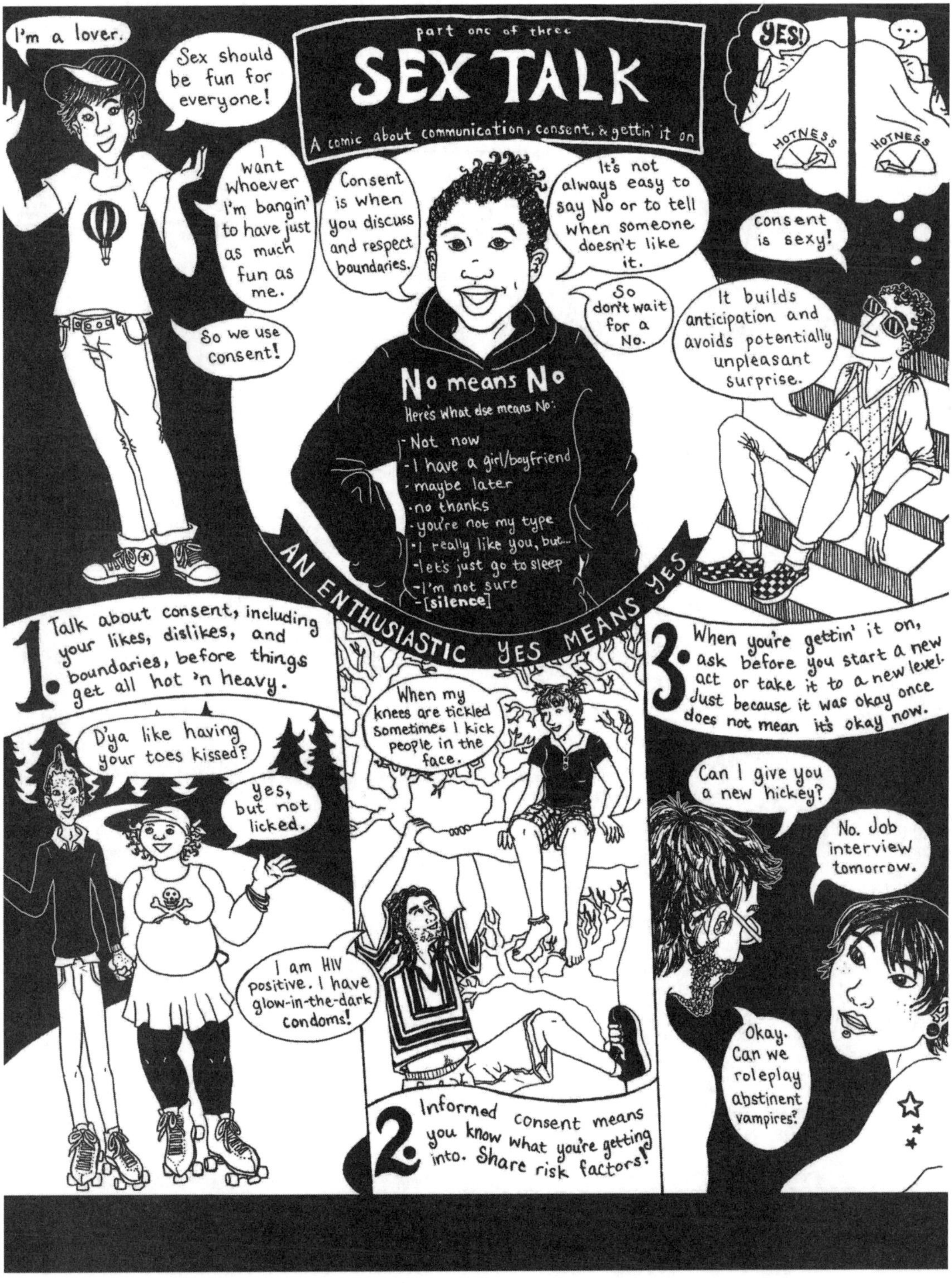

part one of three
SEX TALK
A comic about communication, consent, & gettin' it on
I'm a lover.
Sex should be fun for everyone!
I want whoever I'm bangin' to have just as much fun as me.
So we use consent!
Consent is when you discuss and respect boundaries.
It's not always easy to say No or to tell when someone doesn't like it.
So don't wait for a No.
No means No
Here's what else means No:
- Not now
- I have a girl/boyfriend
- maybe later
- no thanks
- you're not my type
- I really like you, but...
- let's just go to sleep
- I'm not sure
- [silence]
AN ENTHUSIASTIC YES MEANS YES
YES!
HOTNESS
HOTNESS
consent is sexy!
It builds anticipation and avoids potentially unpleasant surprise.
1. Talk about consent, including your likes, dislikes, and boundaries, before things get all hot 'n heavy.
D'ya like having your toes kissed?
Yes, but not licked.
When my knees are tickled sometimes I kick people in the face.
I am HIV positive. I have glow-in-the-dark condoms!
2. Informed consent means you know what you're getting into. Share risk factors!
3. When you're gettin' it on, ask before you start a new act or take it to a new level. Just because it was okay once does not mean it's okay now.
Can I give you a new hickey?
No. Job interview tomorrow.
Okay. Can we roleplay abstinent vampires?

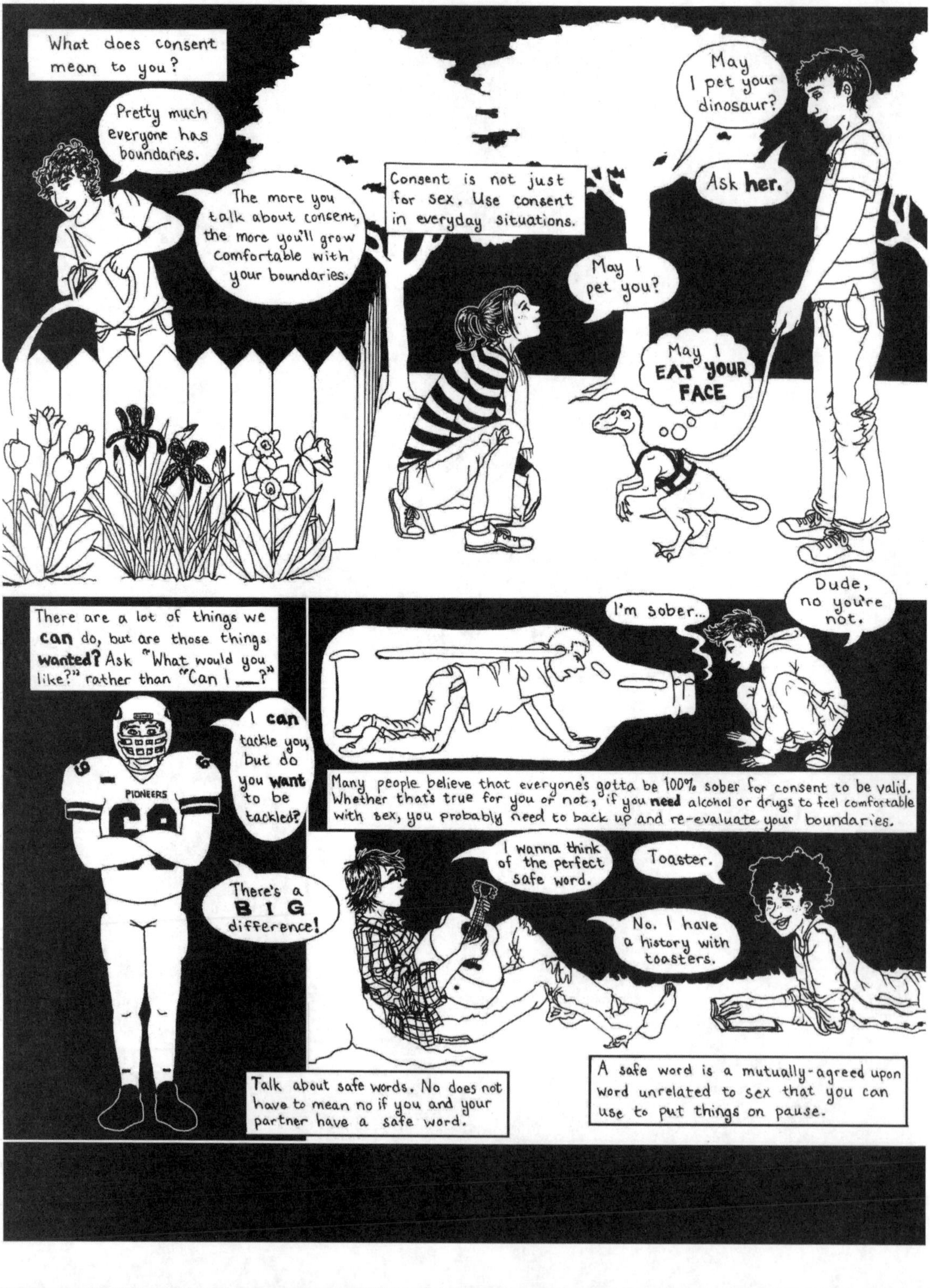

What does consent mean to you?
Pretty much everyone has boundaries.
The more you talk about consent, the more you'll grow comfortable with your boundaries.
Consent is not just for sex. Use consent in everyday situations.
May I pet your dinosaur?
Ask **her.**
May I pet you?
May I **EAT YOUR FACE**
There are a lot of things we **can** do, but are those things **wanted?** Ask "What would you like?" rather than "Can I ___?"
PIONEERS
I **can** tackle you, but do you **want** to be tackled?
There's a **BIG** difference!
I'm sober...
Dude, no you're not.
Many people believe that everyone's gotta be 100% sober for consent to be valid. Whether that's true for you or not, if you **need** alcohol or drugs to feel comfortable with sex, you probably need to back up and re-evaluate your boundaries.
I wanna think of the perfect safe word.
Toaster.
No. I have a history with toasters.
Talk about safe words. No does not have to mean no if you and your partner have a safe word.
A safe word is a mutually-agreed upon word unrelated to sex that you can use to put things on pause.

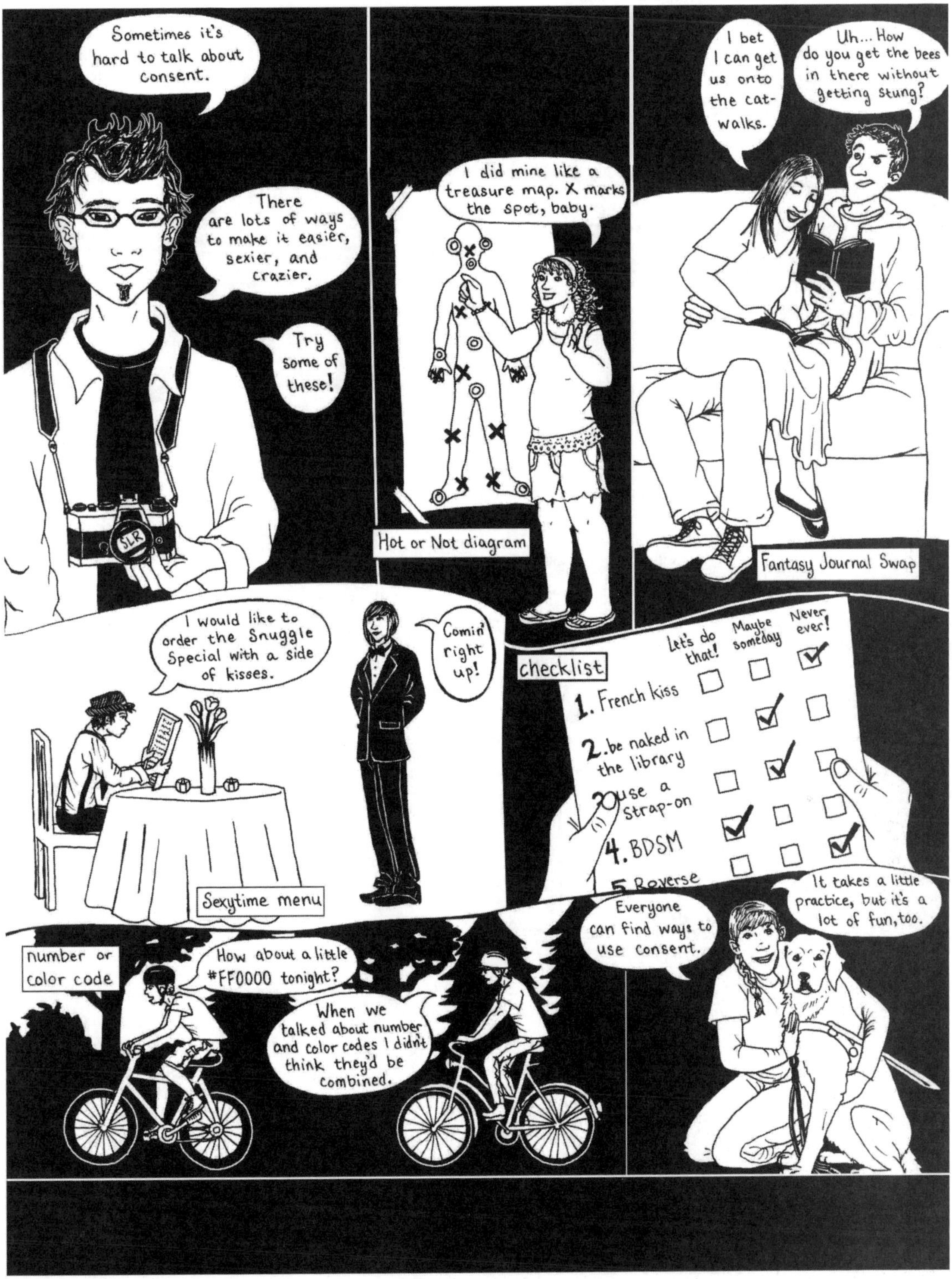
Sometimes it's hard to talk about consent.
There are lots of ways to make it easier, sexier, and crazier.
Try some of these!
SLR
I did mine like a treasure map. X marks the spot, baby.
Hot or Not diagram
I bet I can get us onto the catwalks.
Uh... How do you get the bees in there without getting stung?
Fantasy Journal Swap
I would like to order the Snuggle Special with a side of kisses.
Comin' right up!
Sexytime menu
checklist
Let's do that!
Maybe someday
Never ever!
1. French kiss
2. be naked in the library
3. use a strap-on
4. BDSM
5. Reverse
number or color code
How about a little #FF0000 tonight?
When we talked about number and color codes I didn't think they'd be combined.
Everyone can find ways to use consent.
It takes a little practice, but it's a lot of fun, too.

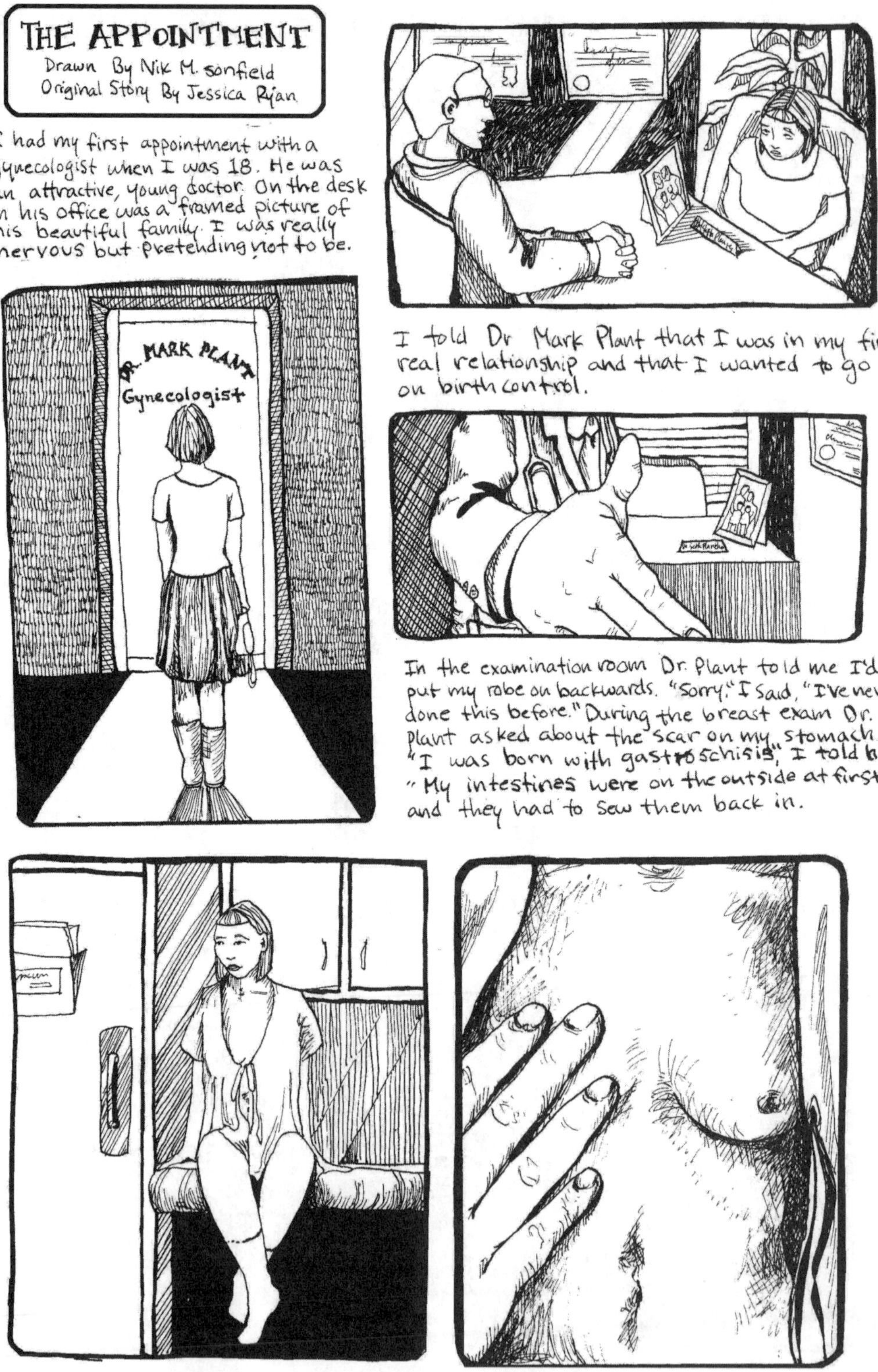
THE APPOINTMENT
Drawn By Nik M. sonfield
Original Story By Jessica Ryan
I had my first appointment with a gynecologist when I was 18. He was an attractive, young doctor. On the desk in his office was a framed picture of his beautiful family. I was really nervous but pretending not to be.
DR. MARK PLANT
Gynecologist
I told Dr Mark Plant that I was in my first real relationship and that I wanted to go on birth control.
In the examination room Dr. Plant told me I'd put my robe on backwards. "Sorry," I said, "I've never done this before." During the breast exam Dr. Plant asked about the scar on my stomach. "I was born with gastroschisis," I told him. "My intestines were on the outside at first and they had to sew them back in.

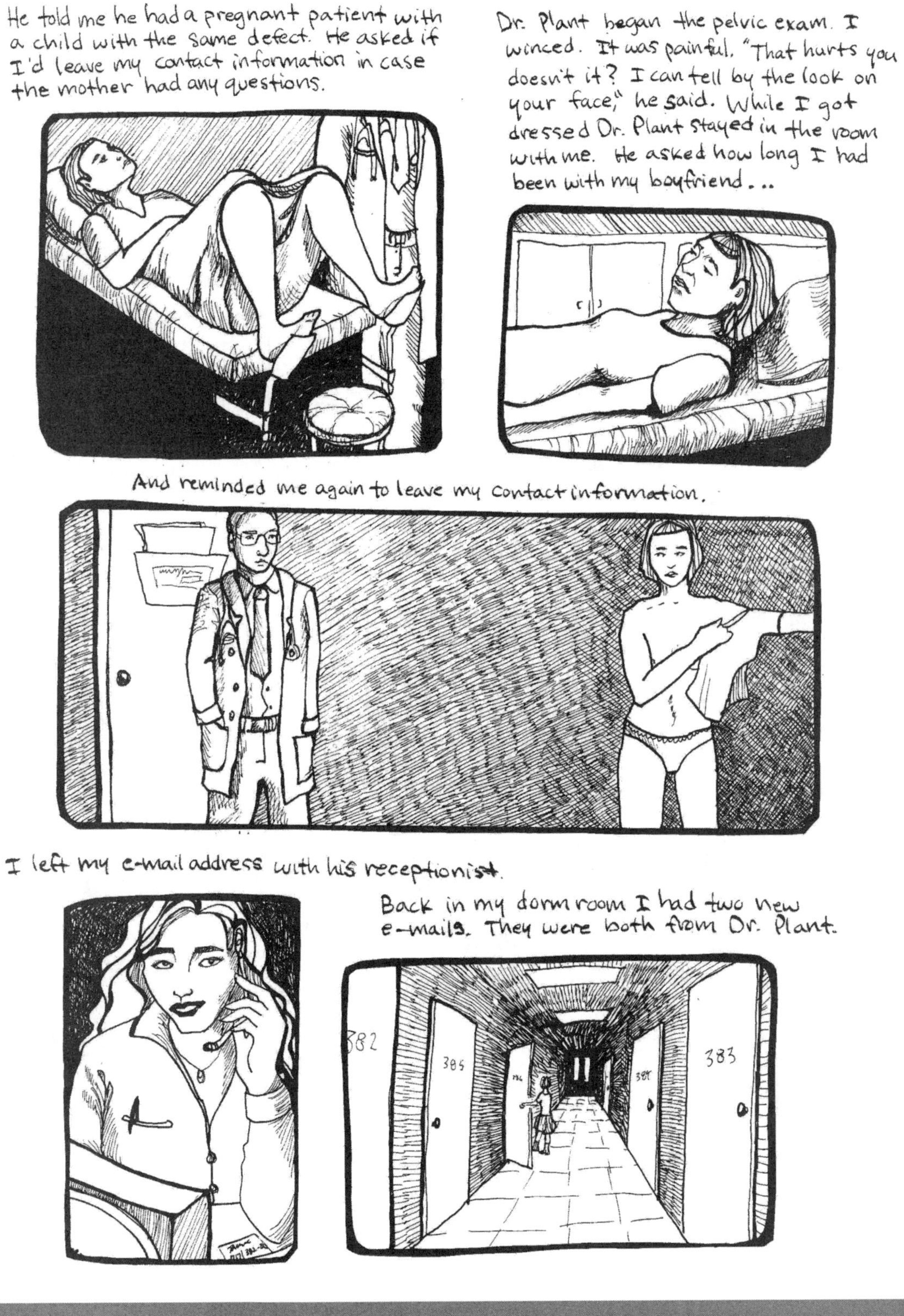
He told me he had a pregnant patient with a child with the same defect. He asked if I'd leave my contact information in case the mother had any questions.
Dr. Plant began the pelvic exam. I winced. It was painful. "That hurts you doesn't it? I can tell by the look on your face," he said. While I got dressed Dr. Plant stayed in the room with me. He asked how long I had been with my boyfriend...
And reminded me again to leave my contact information.
I left my e-mail address with his receptionist.
Back in my dorm room I had two new e-mails. They were both from Dr. Plant.
382
385
383

The first e-mail read...

From: Dr. Mark Plant
To: Agnes M. Smith
Hope you're back in your
and have time
write back.

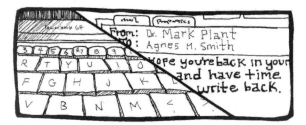

And the second...

It was great meeting today.
I hope we can stay in touch.

The next day there was another e-mail. It said...

Whats your phone number?

I felt sick. There was no pregnant patient. He had lied to me to get my e-mail address. He had watched me change when he should have left the room. He had physically hurt me on purpose. I cried in my room. I felt completely alone.

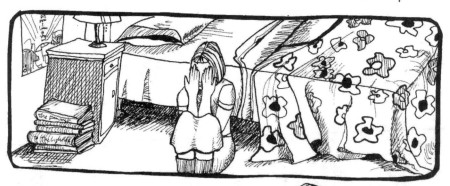

Later I started doing some research. I found sites like Ucomparehealth.com and wrote about my experience so other people would know about Dr. Mark Plant, and so other people could learn from what I had gone through.

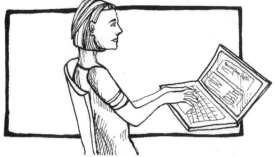

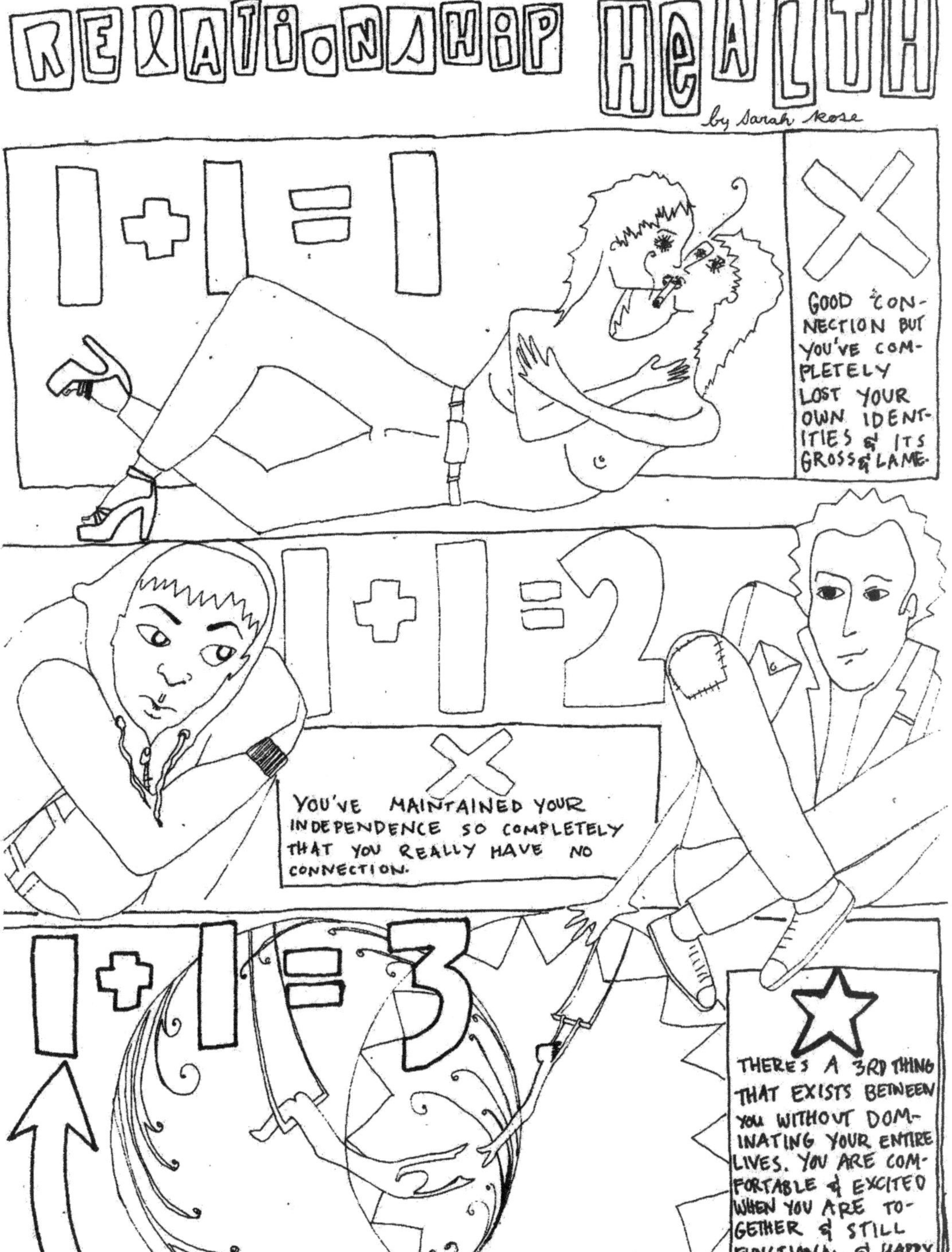
RELATIONSHIP HEALTH
by Sarah Rose
1 + 1 = 1
GOOD CONNECTION BUT YOU'VE COMPLETELY LOST YOUR OWN IDENTITIES & ITS GROSS & LAME.
1 + 1 = 2
YOU'VE MAINTAINED YOUR INDEPENDENCE SO COMPLETELY THAT YOU REALLY HAVE NO CONNECTION.
1 + 1 = 3
THERES A 3RD THING THAT EXISTS BETWEEN YOU WITHOUT DOMINATING YOUR ENTIRE LIVES. YOU ARE COMFORTABLE & EXCITED WHEN YOU ARE TOGETHER & STILL FUNCTIONAL & HAPPY WHEN YOU'RE ALONE.

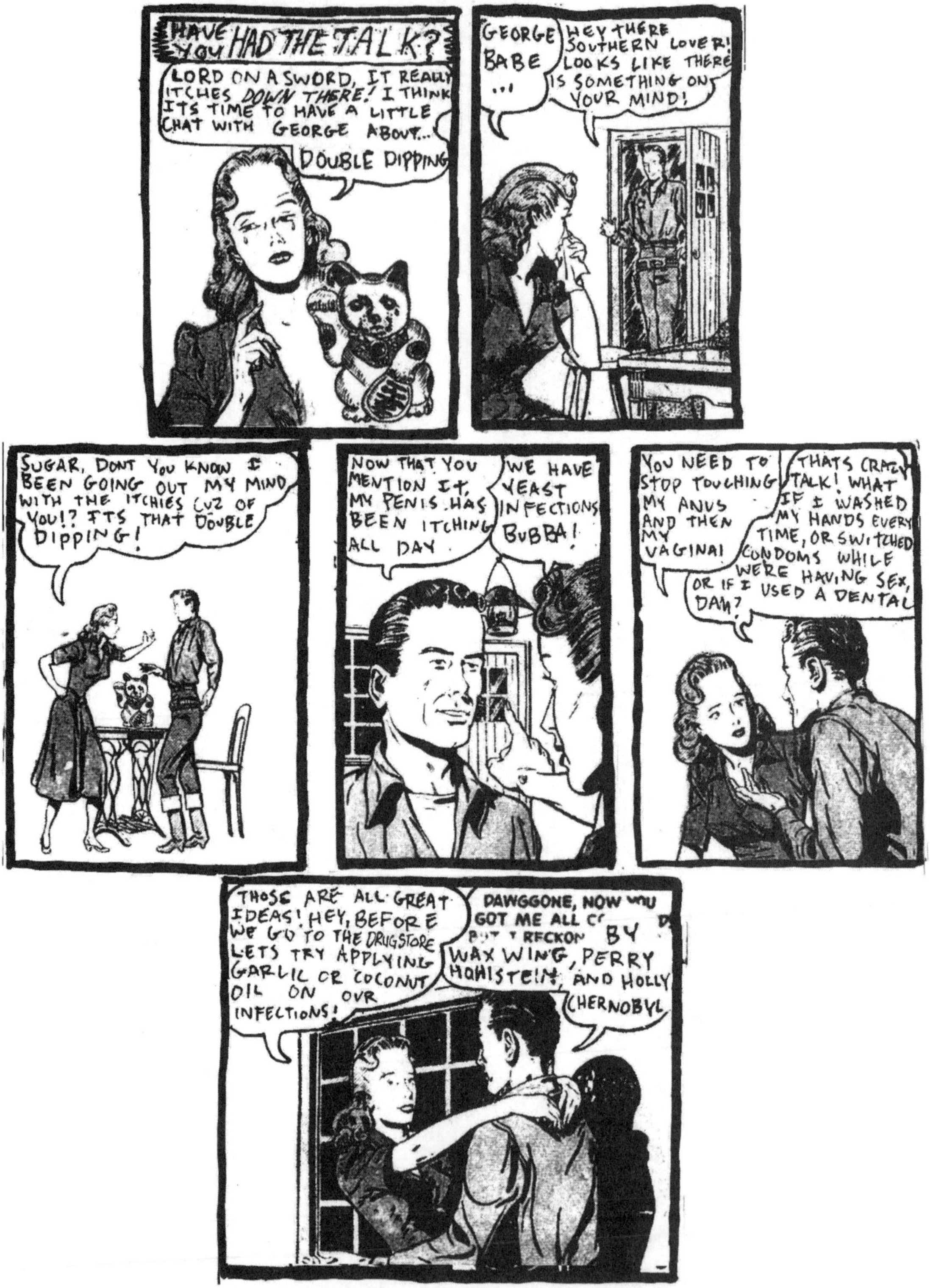
HAVE YOU HAD THE TALK?
LORD ON A SWORD, IT REALLY ITCHES *DOWN THERE!* I THINK ITS TIME TO HAVE A LITTLE CHAT WITH GEORGE ABOUT...
DOUBLE DIPPING
GEORGE BABE ...
HEY THERE SOUTHERN LOVER! LOOKS LIKE THERE IS SOMETHING ON YOUR MIND!
SUGAR, DONT YOU KNOW I BEEN GOING OUT MY MIND WITH THE ITCHIES CUZ OF YOU!? ITS THAT DOUBLE DIPPING!
NOW THAT YOU MENTION IT, MY PENIS HAS BEEN ITCHING ALL DAY
WE HAVE YEAST INFECTIONS BUBBA!
YOU NEED TO STOP TOUCHING MY ANUS AND THEN MY VAGINA!
THATS CRAZY TALK! WHAT IF I WASHED MY HANDS EVERY TIME, OR SWITCHED CONDOMS WHILE WERE HAVING SEX, OR IF I USED A DENTAL DAM?
THOSE ARE ALL GREAT IDEAS! HEY, BEFORE WE GO TO THE DRUGSTORE LETS TRY APPLYING GARLIC OR COCONUT OIL ON OUR INFECTIONS!
DAWGGONE, NOW
GOT ME ALL
BY WAX WING, PERRY HOHLSTEIN, AND HOLLY CHERNOBYL

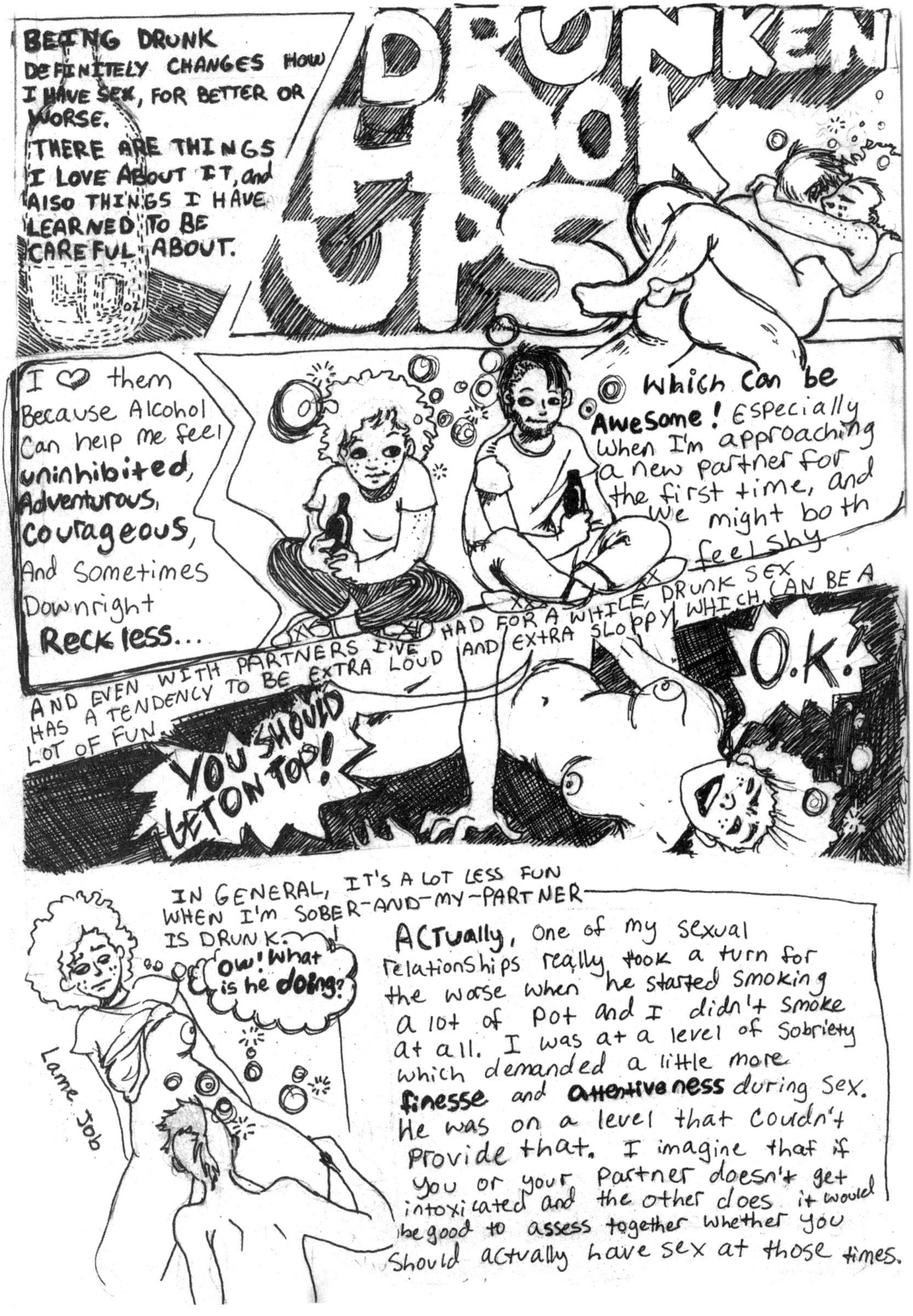

DRUNKEN HOOKUPS
BEING DRUNK DEFINITELY CHANGES HOW I HAVE SEX, FOR BETTER OR WORSE. THERE ARE THINGS I LOVE ABOUT IT, and ALSO THINGS I HAVE LEARNED TO BE CAREFUL ABOUT.
40oz
I ♥ them Because Alcohol can help me feel uninhibited, Adventurous, courageous, And sometimes Downright Reckless...
Which can be Awesome! Especially when I'm approaching a new partner for the first time, and we might both feel shy
AND EVEN WITH PARTNERS I'VE HAD FOR A WHILE, DRUNK SEX HAS A TENDENCY TO BE EXTRA LOUD AND EXTRA SLOPPY, WHICH CAN BE A LOT OF FUN.
YOU SHOULD GET ON TOP!
O.K!
IN GENERAL, IT'S A LOT LESS FUN WHEN I'M SOBER-AND-MY-PARTNER IS DRUNK.
Ow! What is he doing?
Lame Job
ACTually, one of my sexual relationships really took a turn for the worse when he started smoking a lot of pot and I didn't smoke at all. I was at a level of sobriety which demanded a little more finesse and attentiveness during sex. He was on a level that couldn't provide that. I imagine that if you or your partner doesn't get intoxicated and the other does it would be good to assess together whether you should actually have sex at those times.

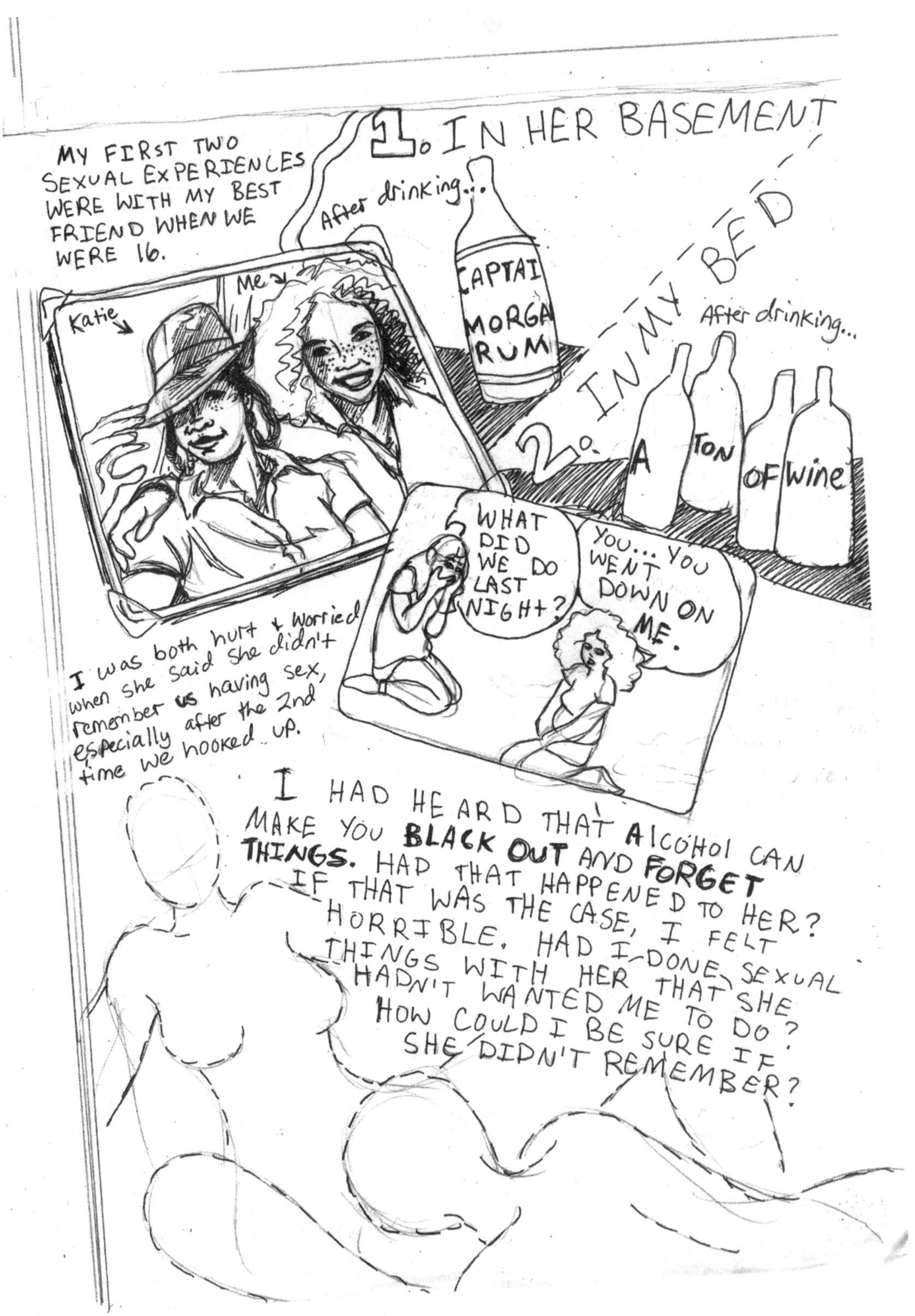
MY FIRST TWO SEXUAL EXPERIENCES WERE WITH MY BEST FRIEND WHEN WE WERE 16.
1. IN HER BASEMENT
After drinking...
CAPTAI MORGA RUM
Me
Katie
2. IN MY BED
After drinking...
A TON OF Wine
WHAT DID WE DO LAST NIGHT?
YOU... YOU WENT DOWN ON ME.
I was both hurt & worried when she said she didn't remember us having sex, especially after the 2nd time we hooked up.
I HAD HEARD THAT ALCOHOL CAN MAKE YOU BLACK OUT AND FORGET THINGS. HAD THAT HAPPENED TO HER? IF THAT WAS THE CASE, I FELT HORRIBLE. HAD I DONE SEXUAL THINGS WITH HER THAT SHE HADN'T WANTED ME TO DO? HOW COULD I BE SURE IF SHE DIDN'T REMEMBER?

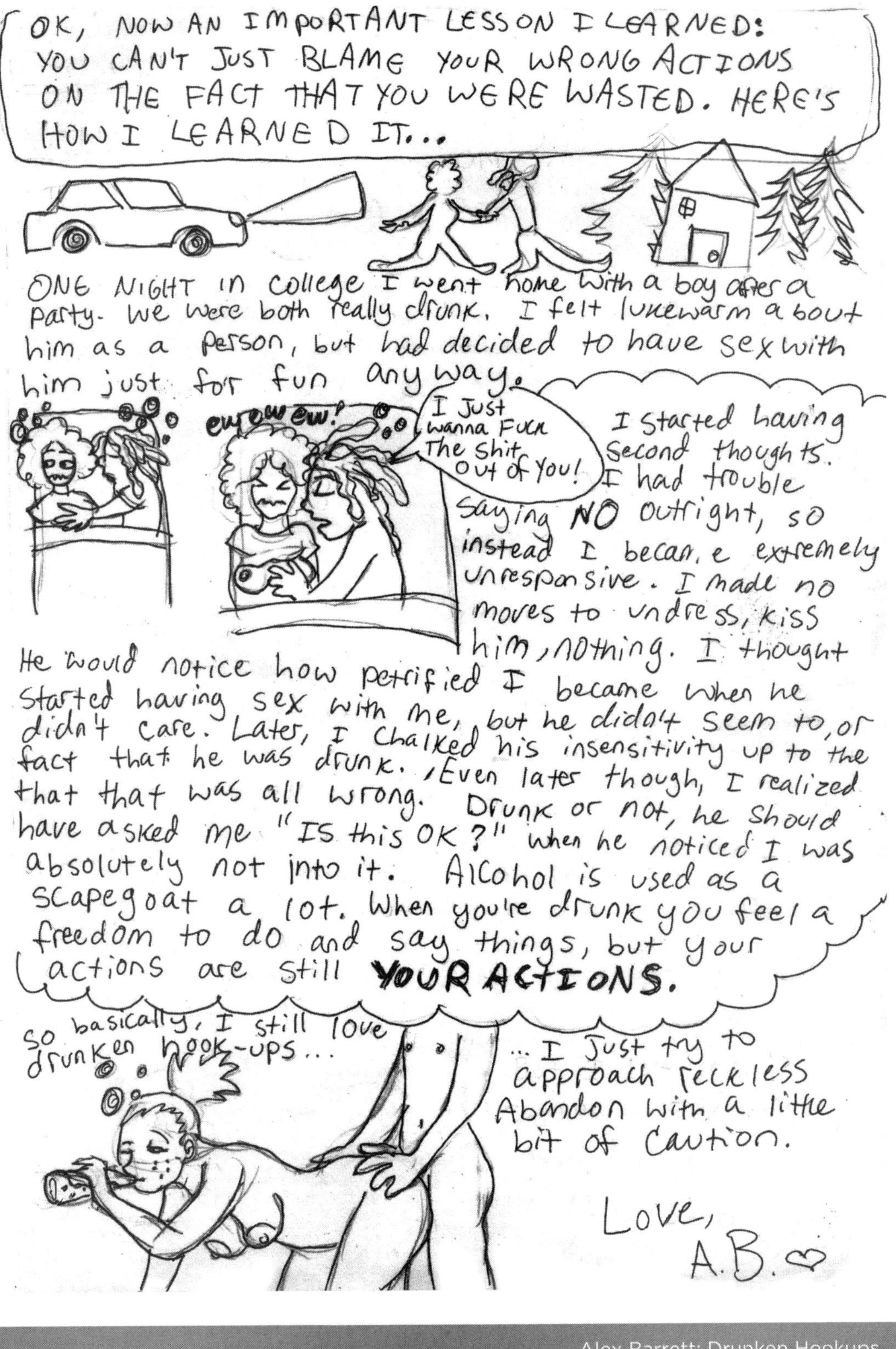
OK, NOW AN IMPORTANT LESSON I LEARNED: YOU CAN'T JUST BLAME YOUR WRONG ACTIONS ON THE FACT THAT YOU WERE WASTED. HERE'S HOW I LEARNED IT...
ONE NIGHT in college I went home with a boy after a party. We were both really drunk. I felt lukewarm about him as a person, but had decided to have sex with him just for fun anyway.
eurewew!
I Just wanna Fuck The shit out of you!
I started having second thoughts. I had trouble saying NO outright, so instead I became extremely unresponsive. I made no moves to undress, kiss him, nothing. I thought he would notice how petrified I became when he started having sex with me, but he didn't seem to, or didn't care. Later, I chalked his insensitivity up to the fact that he was drunk. Even later though, I realized that that was all wrong. Drunk or not, he should have asked me "IS this OK?" when he noticed I was absolutely not into it. Alcohol is used as a scapegoat a lot. When you're drunk you feel a freedom to do and say things, but your actions are still YOUR ACTIONS.
so basically, I still love drunken hook-ups...
...I just try to approach reckless Abandon with a little bit of caution.
Love,
A.B.

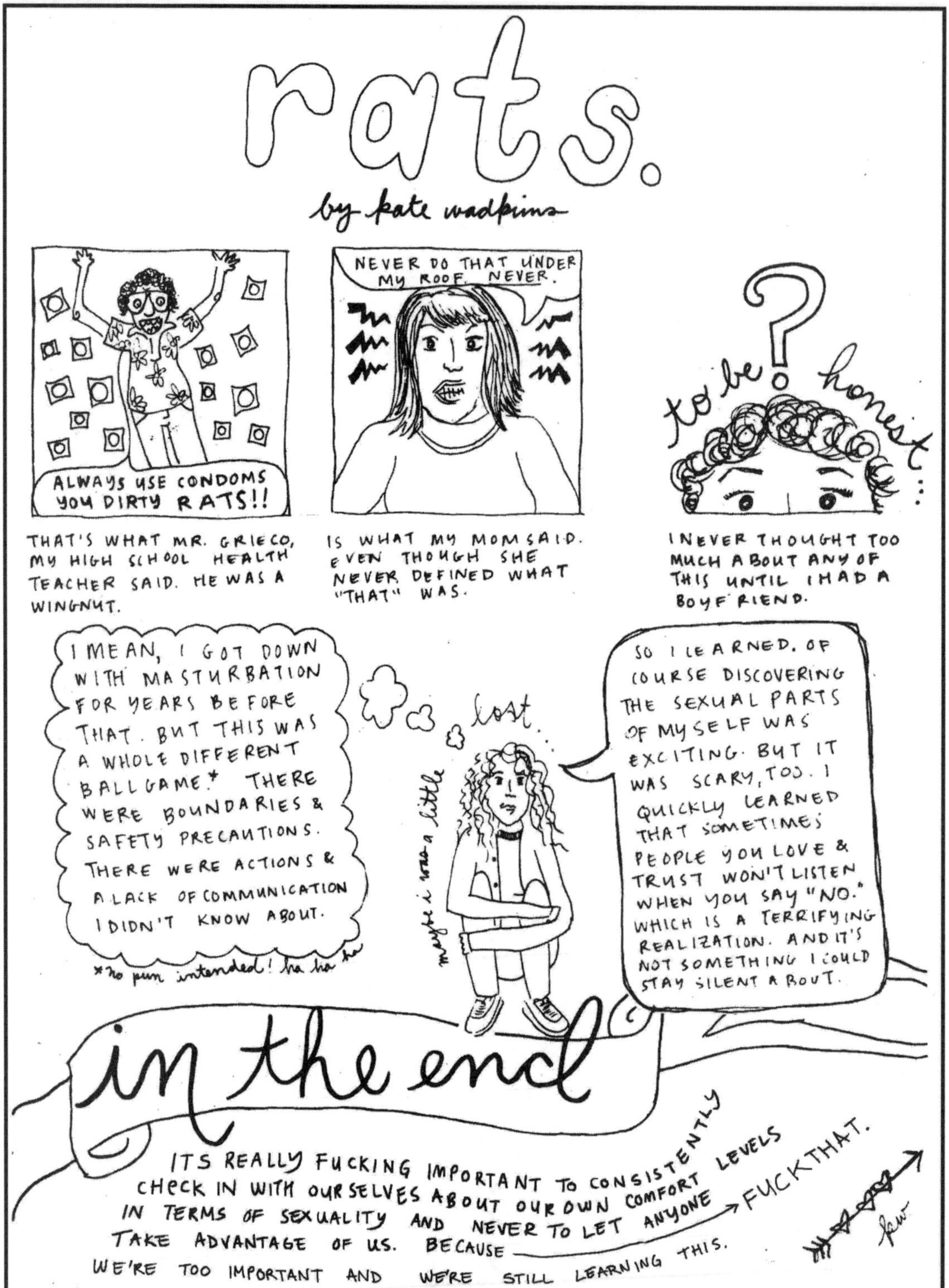
rats.
by kate wadkins
ALWAYS USE CONDOMS YOU DIRTY RATS!!
THAT'S WHAT MR. GRIECO, MY HIGH SCHOOL HEALTH TEACHER SAID. HE WAS A WINGNUT.
NEVER DO THAT UNDER MY ROOF. NEVER.
IS WHAT MY MOM SAID. EVEN THOUGH SHE NEVER DEFINED WHAT "THAT" WAS.
to be honest...
I NEVER THOUGHT TOO MUCH ABOUT ANY OF THIS UNTIL I HAD A BOYFRIEND.
I MEAN, I GOT DOWN WITH MASTURBATION FOR YEARS BEFORE THAT. BUT THIS WAS A WHOLE DIFFERENT BALLGAME.* THERE WERE BOUNDARIES & SAFETY PRECAUTIONS. THERE WERE ACTIONS & A LACK OF COMMUNICATION I DIDN'T KNOW ABOUT.
*no pun intended! ha ha ha
maybe i was a little lost...
SO I LEARNED. OF COURSE DISCOVERING THE SEXUAL PARTS OF MYSELF WAS EXCITING. BUT IT WAS SCARY, TOO. I QUICKLY LEARNED THAT SOMETIMES PEOPLE YOU LOVE & TRUST WON'T LISTEN WHEN YOU SAY "NO." WHICH IS A TERRIFYING REALIZATION. AND IT'S NOT SOMETHING I COULD STAY SILENT ABOUT.
in the end
ITS REALLY FUCKING IMPORTANT TO CONSISTENTLY CHECK IN WITH OURSELVES ABOUT OUR OWN COMFORT LEVELS IN TERMS OF SEXUALITY AND NEVER TO LET ANYONE TAKE ADVANTAGE OF US. BECAUSE WE'RE TOO IMPORTANT AND WE'RE STILL LEARNING THIS.
FUCK THAT.
kw

HAPPY BIRTHDAY

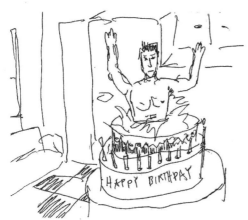

Two years ago today on mister Aaron's birthday
all of manhaus went to the drop in center to test for vd

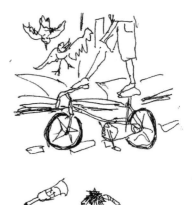

All on bikes so bright and early with plenty of rest
birds were chirping and the air was fresh

CREEPY FEELING

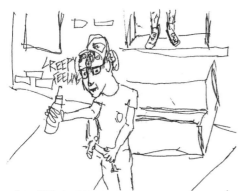

We ran into all kinds of friends along the way
Dan and Andy doing construction on St. Claude drinking O.J.

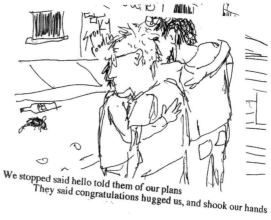

We stopped said hello told them of our plans
They said congratulations hugged us, and shook our hands

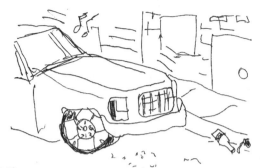

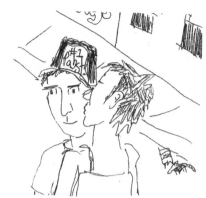

Off we rode once again whistling tunes and wearing grins
We all turned our heads when we heard phat bass
and saw nice rims

Out of nowhere a honk we didn't expect
Our friend Beth stopped and on our cheeks
she did peck

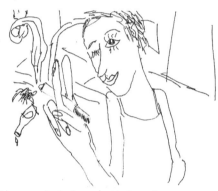

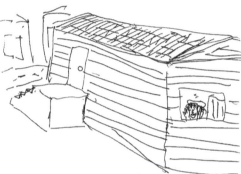

She got excited when we told of our plans
It seemed in the past month she had been with many mans

Along with us she came with her large stride
None else knew last week we hit it in the
double wide

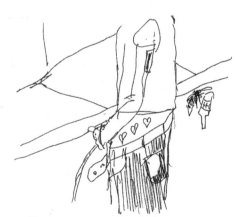

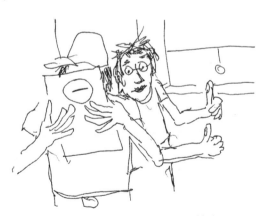

The results of the tests right now I did yearn
For I was starting to think it was Beth that made my pee burn.

We got to the place and waited in line
Aaron and Ethan went in and everything was fine

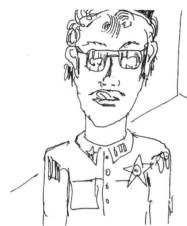

I sat down in the office and my pants I did drop
The doctor felt around on my genitals just like a cop

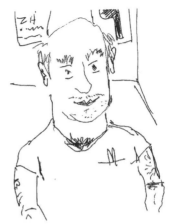

It's no good he said with a very big smile
you won't be having sex for quite a while

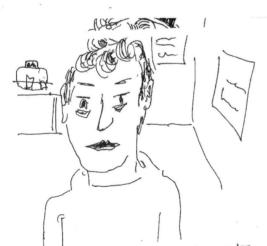

If your scared you can come and sit on my lap
Your not the first boy I've ever met with the clap

EDITOR'S NOTE:
"THE CLAP" = GONORRHEA
AND IS
EASILY
TREATABLE!

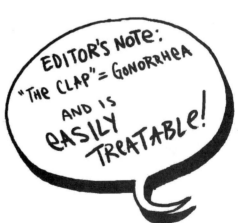

CHAPTER FOUR:

IDENTITY

LIZA

Prospects of my own sexuality have excited me since the long recesses at Miss Tucker's Montessori School. Selfish needs of wanting to be desired by my peers—girls and boys alike—led to games of chasing the other children around trying to kiss them.

If I sought out desire in preschool, this need only intensified during elementary school. I was bullied often and cruelly, which only increased my need to be liked and accepted. I was teased for the things I said, the clothes I wore, the games I liked to play, my hair, the way I mixed up words when I read, and anything else that seemed odd to the rest of the girls. Their cruelness ate at me throughout the rest of my life, but I never felt that I was in the wrong. I continued to wear, say, and do "weird" things. However, there was one experience that raised lasting insecurities.

From the second to fourth grade I carpooled with a classmate. We also participated in extracurricular activities together. We saw a lot of each other. My mother dropped me at her house in the mornings before school. I waited in the living room as both she and her mother got ready for the day. One morning my friend said, "I'm going to change my clothes. Don't watch me through the crack in my wall."

I hadn't even known there was a crack in her wall. I sat on that couch every morning watching TV and never noticed it. But there it was: a split in the wall a quarter inch wide. Could I really see anything through it? I absolutely had to peek. I saw her standing, still wearing her pajamas, staring at me from the other side of the crack.

MY FIRST TIME IN A RELATIONSHIP TYPE THING WITH A GIRL
ME
HER
IT WAS FUN!
UNTIL IT WASN'T...
NEW VOICE MAIL
LIZA, WE NEED TO... TALK

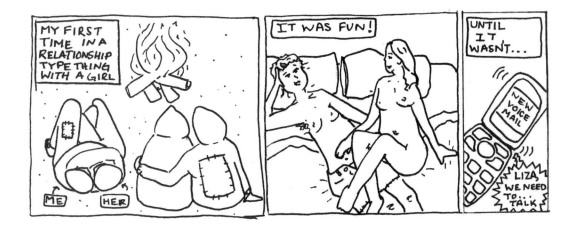

"You looked! You are sick!"

Once we got to school, it took five minutes for the news of this event to spread. Girls pretended to be uncomfortable around me because now I was gay and gross. I was teased throughout the day, but then, I was teased most days. The difference here was that I felt guilty: even though my friend had specifically told me not to look, I had looked. When my mother arrived to take us home, my friend was still angry. I didn't have the words to apologize in a way that would make her understand.

SAIYA

In the house where I grew up, there was a room full of dress-up clothes. It had an ugly brown carpet and lacy curtains, and there were trunks lining the wall, bursting with old dresses, suits, silk scarves, and hats. This is where my brother and I spent most of our childhood, and where I learned the art of drag. There are pictures of us with grave expressions on our faces, dressed as two waitresses. Medieval serfs and peasants were a source of endless inspiration. There was a blue shirt with gold buttons that could belong to a policeman or a sailor, depending on our mood. My brother was the guinea pig for all of my experiments regarding which clothes made women and which made men. I once dressed him as Little Bo Peep and made him sit behind our lemonade stand while I hid behind a tree and tallied up the number of customers who thought he was a girl. I remember thinking that it was scary, how seriously everyone else seemed to feel about the game of dress-up. I saw the grown-ups shaking their heads and chuckling nervously. I knew we only got away with it because we were kids.

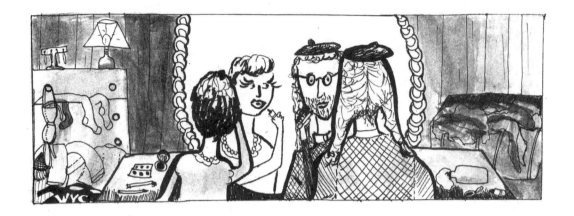

Not much later, I would go into the room alone and close the door. I carefully calculated the place in the room where no one would be able to see me through either of the windows or the doorway, and tried putting my hands between my legs. The terror of someone finding me was only partially blocked out by the urgent need to try this. Then the room became different, exciting and bad at the same time. I would find musty old stockings and pair them with ties that smelled like cologne. There was something forbidden about certain clothing, some secret in them that I could only learn by putting them on and then taking them off.

AT SOME POINT I STARTED using clothing as a defense mechanism. I had a rotating selection of special pieces of clothing, and they became my armor. Each fit my body perfectly because it had been worn into my shape over time. When something went missing, I felt naked on the street. A scenario would unfold that went something like this: *Oh no, where is my hat? No no no no, this isn't happening. I think I lost my hat. I don't want to wear that other hat; I need MY hat! My special hat, the green one with the brown ear flaps. The one I always wear.*

I want to believe I could feel prepared to face the street wearing any old thing. In fact, I like to experiment with this, and sometimes dress myself up as a pinup starlet or a business lady and watch the world see me differently. I watch other people closely and mimic them in their costumes, imitating the way they move in their clothes.

I adorn my body carefully, because it affects how I carry myself. I hold on to a little metal horseshoe when I miss my old friend who gave it to me. I have a good luck coin with a hole through it, and it really works. The things I string around my neck protect me. My hair is a big part of this also. I use it as I go, pulling it back and out of my face when I feel serious and I need to get things done quickly, braiding it intently, playing with its crazy shapes and letting it fly in the wind, letting it curl around me when I have something secret going on, pulling up my hood when I am angry, sad, and cold.

I often want to look like a boy, but it is rarely possible. I have real hips and huge hair and everything else. Instead, I have my own version of masculinity; I know it is there even when it is invisible to everyone else. I like to make my own way, choosing what to wear and seeing how it feels. Sometimes I end up looking like a little kid who got dressed with her eyes closed, which is okay. I craft my own suit of armor for each day, finding it boring to choose between only two genders. I have too many cool outfits.

LIZA

My affairs with cisgender men were always the easiest to navigate. While they were not healthy or free of manipulation, I at least had a road map for them. There was a simple narrative to follow. It was not just about flirting. When I felt attracted to a man, I knew what to say and how to assess his actions. There was no mystery or fear that I was acting inappropriately. The culture of heteronormativity contributes to this ease. Disappointment and rejection are part of the experience, but not unexpected. Heterosexual stories of attraction, romance, and rejection are pervasively privileged by media and mainstream recounted histories.

Women are more intimidating. There is a fear, homophobia, inside me. Guilt. I do not have a narrative to follow, except shame. After breaking up with my high school boyfriend, I started to explore the idea of intimacy with women: first alone, then with porn, then in dark corners at bars. Beginning love with a woman shakes my core. Beyond the adrenalin of having new partners and new sex, it feels like confronting that childhood fear and guilt.

As a queer woman I feel like my gayness is under constant attack. The worst, and possibly only, challenger is myself. I feel guilty if I'm attracted to a man because I'm implicit in the heteronormative narrative. I am afraid to initiate a partnership with a woman because I'm worried she will think I am too straight. I used to think my queerness would erase the binary completely, but instead it can intensify it, stunting my romantic attempts.

SAIYA

In high school science class, we learned about solids and liquids and gases. To demonstrate just how slight the differences between them can be, we mixed water with cornstarch, making a messy white glob on each of our desks and poking at it. Something bizarre happened. If you put pressure on the blob and squeezed it in your hand, it compressed into a solid shape. Then, as soon as you released your force upon it, it melted, oozing through your fingers and dripping back onto the desk. I was mesmerized. The teacher's voice became muted in the background as she moved on to explain the mathematical formula behind this phenomenon, but I could not stop clenching and unclenching my fist around the blob, watching it take shape and then dissolve. I knew how it felt to be able to hold shape like that, to pose when squeezed, and then to melt away, formless, when given the chance.

The youth of today may tend to be more fluid in their identities and resistant to labels and boxes. Therefore, it is important that sex education includes discussions that were previously reserved only for "gay kids" and vice versa; assumptions that associate certain types of anatomy with certain types of sex can be inaccurate and dangerous. Many teenagers now have multiple partners, multiple genders, and a variety of sexual orientations. Sex education needs to be about managing more than just the mechanics. This means more focus on discussing relationships, emotions, and confusion. The mechanics that are taught, however, need to be learned by everyone.

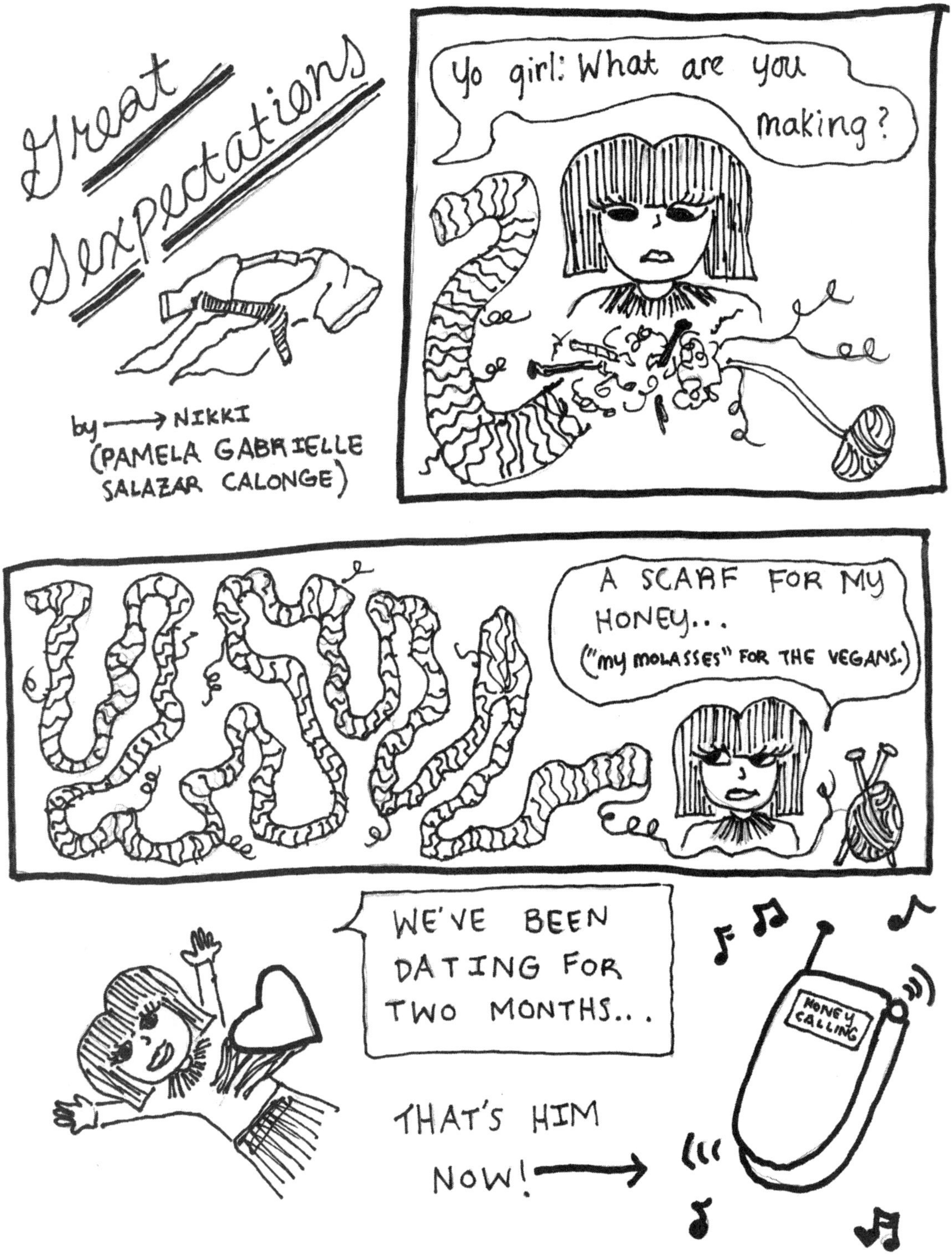

Great Sexpectations
by → NIKKI (PAMELA GABRIELLE SALAZAR CALONGE)
Yo girl: What are you making?
A SCARF FOR MY HONEY... ("my MOLASSES" FOR THE VEGANS.)
WE'VE BEEN DATING FOR TWO MONTHS...
THAT'S HIM NOW! →
HONEY CALLING

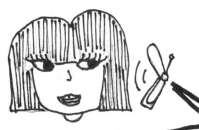
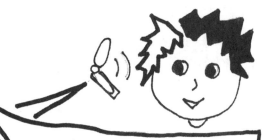

YOU WANT TO SWITCH GIFTS TONIGHT?

WHAT A GOOD IDEA! (OOOOO TONIGHT...)

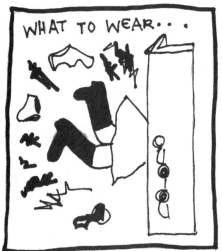

WHAT TO WEAR...

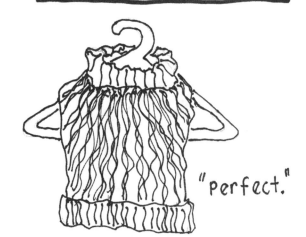

"perfect."

TWO HOURS LATER ...

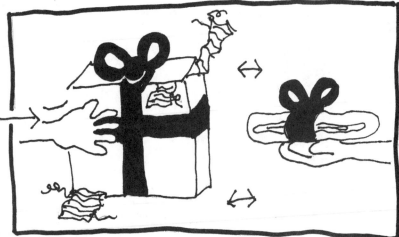

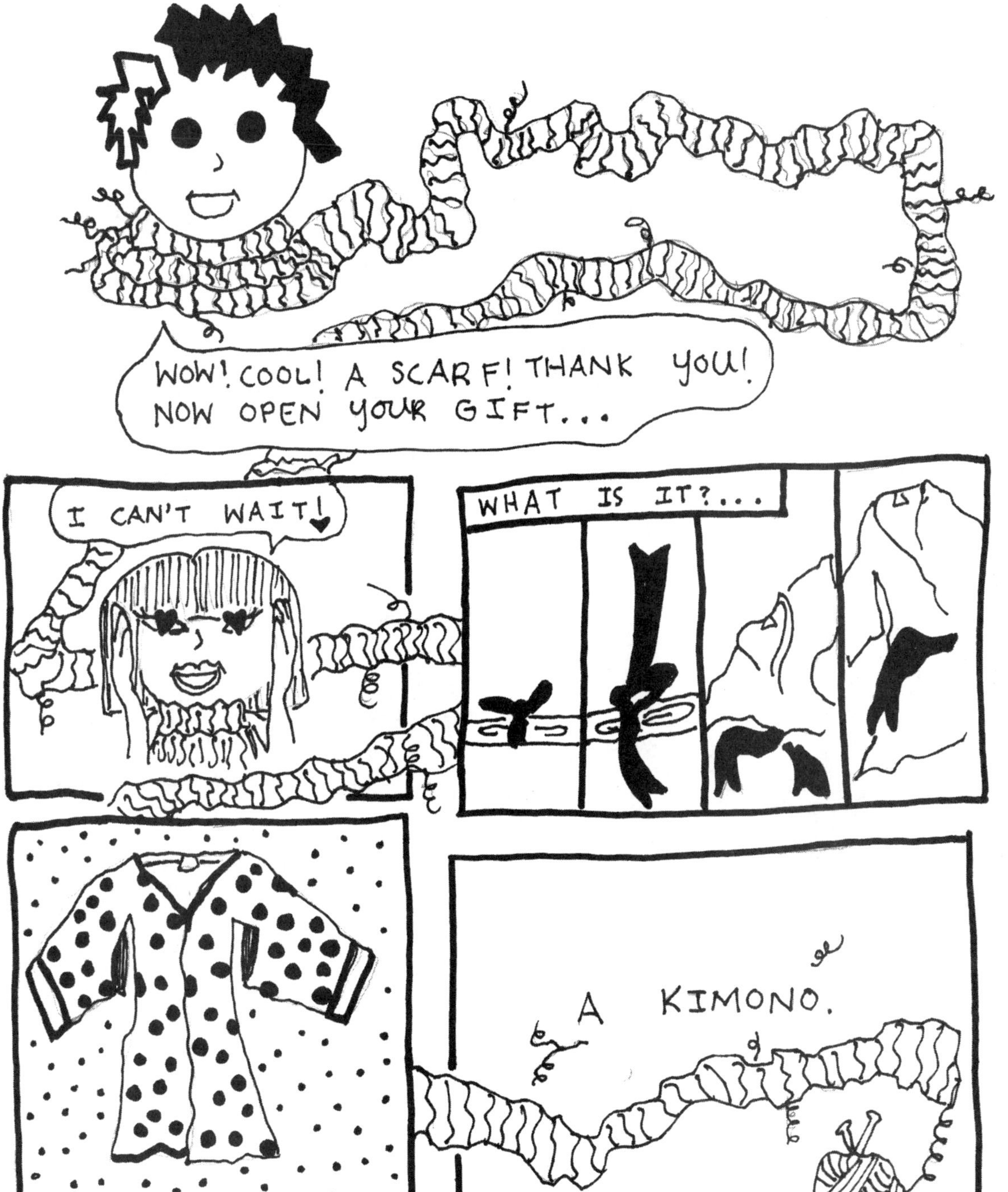
WOW! COOL! A SCARF! THANK YOU! NOW OPEN YOUR GIFT...
I CAN'T WAIT!
WHAT IS IT?...
A KIMONO.
A KIMONO.

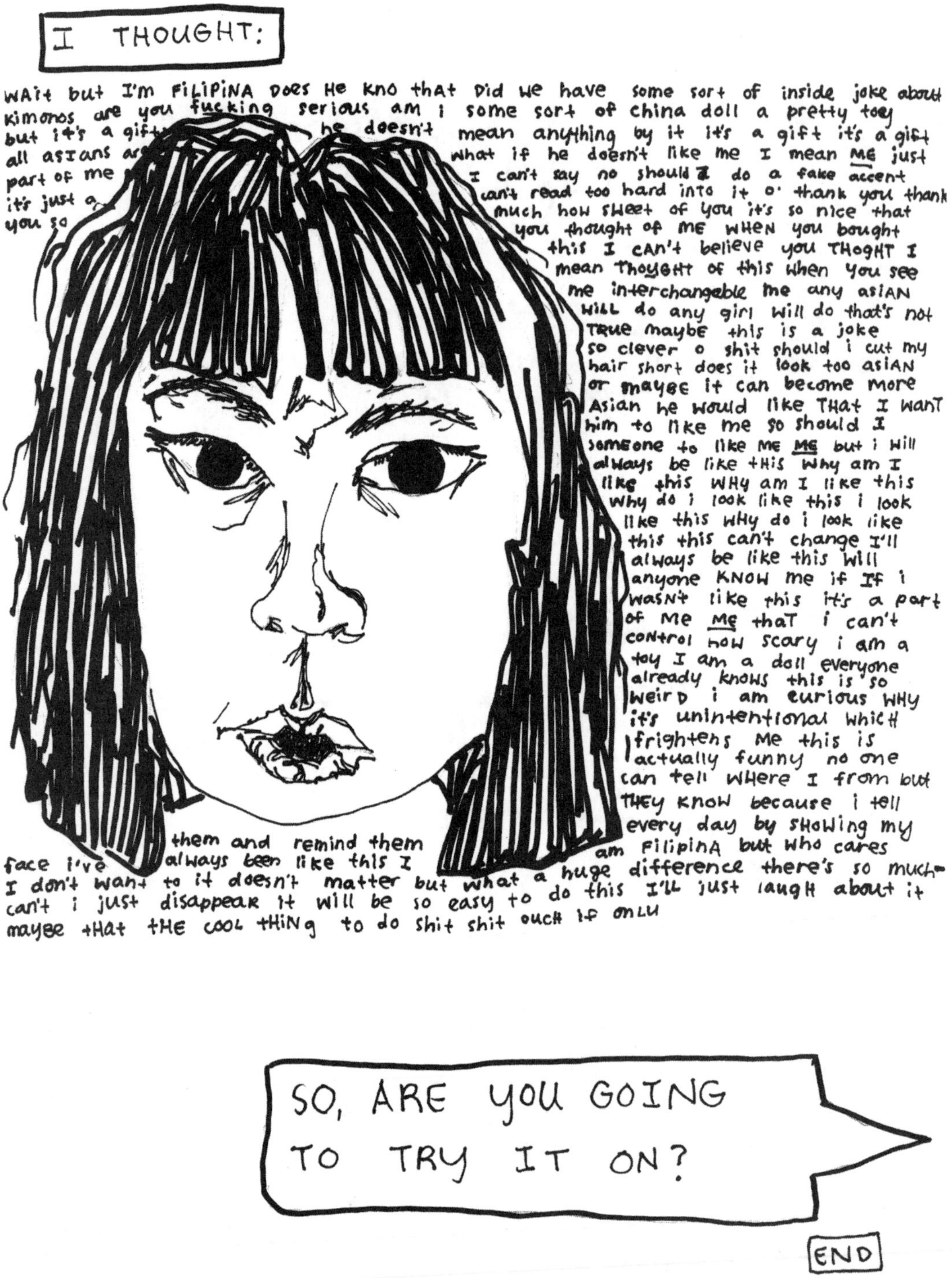
I THOUGHT:
WAit but I'm FILIPINA Does He kno that Did we have some sort of inside joke about
kimonos are you fucking serious am i some sort of china doll a pretty toey
but it's a gift
he doesn't mean anything by it it's a gift it's a gift
all asIans ar
what if he doesn't like me I mean ME just
part of me
I can't say no should I do a fake accent
it's just a
can't read too hard into it o' thank you thank
you so
much how sweet of you it's so nice that
you thought of ME WHEN you bought
this I cAN't believe you THOgHT I
mean ThoyGHT of this when You see
me interchangeable me any asIAN
WILL do any girl will do that's not
TRUE maybE this is a joke
so clever o shit should i cut my
hair short does it look too asIAN
or mayBE it can become more
Asian he would like THat I WanT
him to like me so should I
someone to like ME ME but i will
always be like tHis why am I
like this WHy am I like this
why do i look like this i look
like this wHy do i look like
this this can't change I'll
always be like this will
anyone KNOW me if If i
wasn't like this it's a part
of Me ME thaT i can't
control how scary i am a
toy I am a doll everyone
already knows this is so
weirD i am curious WHY
it's unintentional whicH
frightens Me this is
actually funny no one
can tell WHere I from but
THEY KNOW because i tell
every day by sHoWing my
them and remind them
am FilipinA but who cares
face i've
always been like this I
what a huge difference there's so much
I don't want to it doesn't matter but
can't i just disappear it will be so easy to do this I'll just laugh about it
maybe tHat tHE cooL tHiNg to do shit shit ouch if onlu
SO, ARE YOU GOING TO TRY IT ON?
END

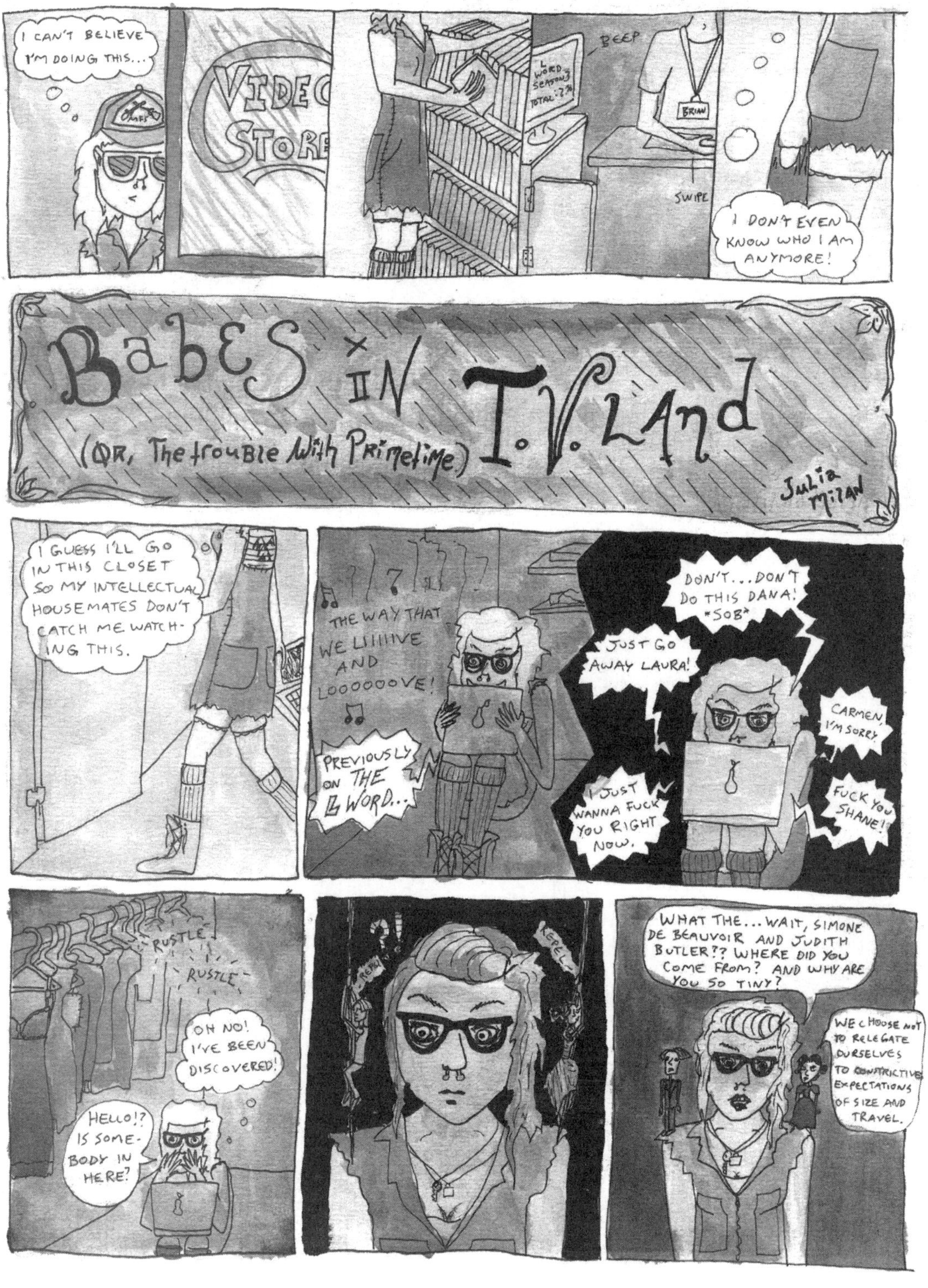

I CAN'T BELIEVE I'M DOING THIS...
VIDEO STORE
BEEP
L WORD SEASON 3 TOTAL: 2?
BRIAN
SWIPE
I DON'T EVEN KNOW WHO I AM ANYMORE!
Babes in T.V. Land
(OR, The trouble With Primetime)
Julia Milan
I GUESS I'LL GO IN THIS CLOSET SO MY INTELLECTUAL HOUSEMATES DON'T CATCH ME WATCHING THIS.
THE WAY THAT WE LIIIIIVE AND LOOOOOOVE!
PREVIOUSLY ON THE L WORD...
DON'T... DON'T DO THIS DANA! *SOB*
JUST GO AWAY LAURA!
CARMEN, I'M SORRY.
I JUST WANNA FUCK YOU RIGHT NOW.
FUCK YOU SHANE!
RUSTLE
RUSTLE
OH NO! I'VE BEEN DISCOVERED!
HELLO!? IS SOMEBODY IN HERE?
REPEL
REPEL
WHAT THE... WAIT, SIMONE DE BEAUVOIR AND JUDITH BUTLER?? WHERE DID YOU COME FROM? AND WHY ARE YOU SO TINY?
WE CHOOSE NOT TO RELEGATE OURSELVES TO CONSTRICTIVE EXPECTATIONS OF SIZE AND TRAVEL.

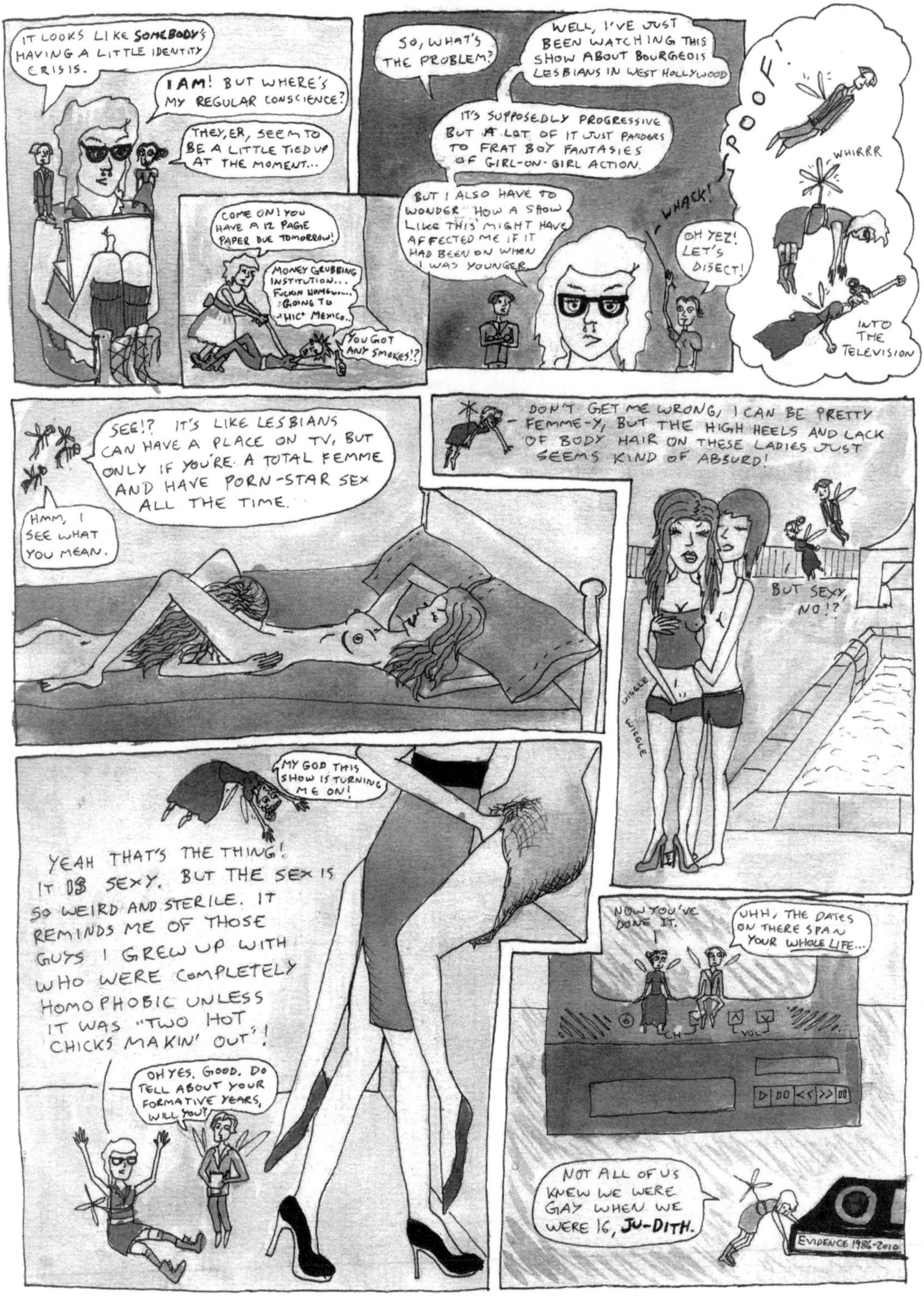
IT LOOKS LIKE SOMEBODY'S HAVING A LITTLE IDENTITY CRISIS.
I AM! BUT WHERE'S MY REGULAR CONSCIENCE?
THEY, ER, SEEM TO BE A LITTLE TIED UP AT THE MOMENT...
COME ON! YOU HAVE A 12 PAGE PAPER DUE TOMORROW!
MONEY GRUBBING INSTITUTION... FUCKIN HOMEW... GOING TO *HIC* MEXICO..
YOU GOT ANY SMOKES!?
SO, WHAT'S THE PROBLEM?
WELL, I'VE JUST BEEN WATCHING THIS SHOW ABOUT BOURGEOIS LESBIANS IN WEST HOLLYWOOD
IT'S SUPPOSEDLY PROGRESSIVE BUT A LOT OF IT JUST PANDERS TO FRAT BOY FANTASIES OF GIRL-ON-GIRL ACTION.
BUT I ALSO HAVE TO WONDER HOW A SHOW LIKE THIS MIGHT HAVE AFFECTED ME IF IT HAD BEEN ON WHEN I WAS YOUNGER.
WHACK!
OH YEZ! LET'S DISECT!
POOF!
WHIRRR
INTO THE TELEVISION
SEE!? IT'S LIKE LESBIANS CAN HAVE A PLACE ON TV, BUT ONLY IF YOU'RE A TOTAL FEMME AND HAVE PORN-STAR SEX ALL THE TIME.
HMM, I SEE WHAT YOU MEAN.
DON'T GET ME WRONG, I CAN BE PRETTY FEMME-Y, BUT THE HIGH HEELS AND LACK OF BODY HAIR ON THESE LADIES JUST SEEMS KIND OF ABSURD!
BUT SEXY, NO!?
WIGGLE WIGGLE
MY GOD THIS SHOW IS TURNING ME ON!
YEAH THAT'S THE THING! IT IS SEXY. BUT THE SEX IS SO WEIRD AND STERILE. IT REMINDS ME OF THOSE GUYS I GREW UP WITH WHO WERE COMPLETELY HOMOPHOBIC UNLESS IT WAS "TWO HOT CHICKS MAKIN' OUT"!
OH YES. GOOD. DO TELL ABOUT YOUR FORMATIVE YEARS, WILL YOU?
NOW YOU'VE DONE IT.
UHH, THE DATES ON THERE SPAN YOUR WHOLE LIFE...
CH
VOL
NOT ALL OF US KNEW WE WERE GAY WHEN WE WERE 16, JU-DITH.
EVIDENCE 1986-2010

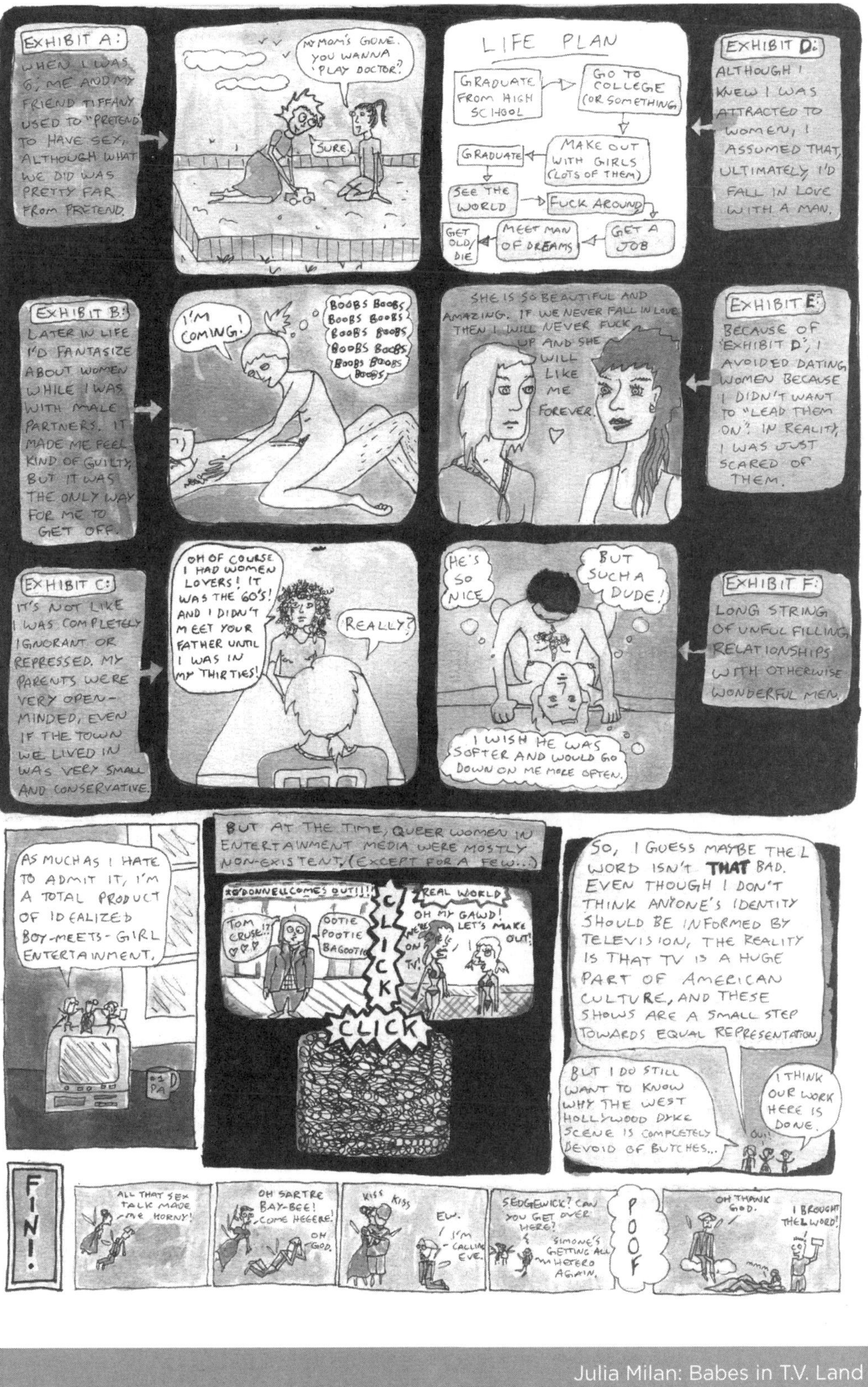
EXHIBIT A:
WHEN I WAS 6, ME AND MY FRIEND TIFFANY USED TO "PRETEND" TO HAVE SEX, ALTHOUGH WHAT WE DID WAS PRETTY FAR FROM PRETEND.
MY MOM'S GONE. YOU WANNA 'PLAY DOCTOR'?
SURE.
LIFE PLAN
GRADUATE FROM HIGH SCHOOL
GO TO COLLEGE (OR SOMETHING)
MAKE OUT WITH GIRLS (LOTS OF THEM)
GRADUATE
SEE THE WORLD
FUCK AROUND
GET A JOB
MEET MAN OF DREAMS
GET OLD/ DIE
EXHIBIT D:
ALTHOUGH I KNEW I WAS ATTRACTED TO WOMEN, I ASSUMED THAT, ULTIMATELY, I'D FALL IN LOVE WITH A MAN.
EXHIBIT B:
LATER IN LIFE I'D FANTASIZE ABOUT WOMEN WHILE I WAS WITH MALE PARTNERS. IT MADE ME FEEL KIND OF GUILTY, BUT IT WAS THE ONLY WAY FOR ME TO GET OFF.
I'M COMING!
BOOBS BOOBS BOOBS BOOBS BOOBS BOOBS BOOBS BOOBS BOOBS BOOBS BOOBS
SHE IS SO BEAUTIFUL AND AMAZING. IF WE NEVER FALL IN LOVE THEN I WILL NEVER FUCK UP AND SHE WILL LIKE ME FOREVER.
EXHIBIT E:
BECAUSE OF 'EXHIBIT D', I AVOIDED DATING WOMEN BECAUSE I DIDN'T WANT TO "LEAD THEM ON". IN REALITY, I WAS JUST SCARED OF THEM.
EXHIBIT C:
IT'S NOT LIKE I WAS COMPLETELY IGNORANT OR REPRESSED. MY PARENTS WERE VERY OPEN-MINDED, EVEN IF THE TOWN WE LIVED IN WAS VERY SMALL AND CONSERVATIVE.
OH OF COURSE I HAD WOMEN LOVERS! IT WAS THE 60'S! AND I DIDN'T MEET YOUR FATHER UNTIL I WAS IN MY THIRTIES!
REALLY?
HE'S SO NICE
BUT SUCH A DUDE!
I WISH HE WAS SOFTER AND WOULD GO DOWN ON ME MORE OFTEN.
EXHIBIT F:
LONG STRING OF UNFULFILLING RELATIONSHIPS WITH OTHERWISE WONDERFUL MEN.
AS MUCH AS I HATE TO ADMIT IT, I'M A TOTAL PRODUCT OF IDEALIZED BOY-MEETS-GIRL ENTERTAINMENT.
BUT AT THE TIME, QUEER WOMEN IN ENTERTAINMENT MEDIA WERE MOSTLY NON-EXISTENT. (EXCEPT FOR A FEW...)
O'DONNELL COMES OUT!!!
TOM CRUSE!?
OOTIE POOTIE BAGOOTIE
CLICK
REAL WORLD
OH MY GAWD! WE'RE ON TV!
LET'S MAKE OUT!
CLICK
SO, I GUESS MAYBE THE L WORD ISN'T THAT BAD. EVEN THOUGH I DON'T THINK ANYONE'S IDENTITY SHOULD BE INFORMED BY TELEVISION, THE REALITY IS THAT TV IS A HUGE PART OF AMERICAN CULTURE, AND THESE SHOWS ARE A SMALL STEP TOWARDS EQUAL REPRESENTATION.
BUT I DO STILL WANT TO KNOW WHY THE WEST HOLLYWOOD DYKE SCENE IS COMPLETELY DEVOID OF BUTCHES...
I THINK OUR WORK HERE IS DONE.
OUI!
FINI.
ALL THAT SEX TALK MADE ME HORNY!
OH SARTRE BAY-BEE! COME HEEERE!
OH GOD.
KISS KISS
EW.
I'M CALLING EVE.
SEDGEWICK? CAN YOU GET OVER HERE?
SIMONE'S GETTING ALL HETERO AGAIN.
POOF
OH THANK GOD.
I BROUGHT THE L WORD!

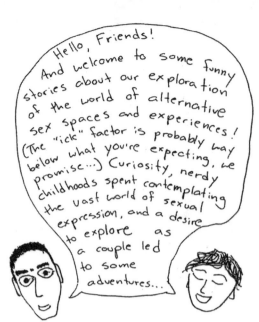

Hello, Friends! And welcome to some funny stories about our exploration of the world of alternative sex spaces and experiences! (The "ick" factor is probably way below what you're expecting, we promise...) Curiosity, nerdy childhoods spent contemplating the vast world of sexual expression, and a desire to explore as a couple led to some adventures...

As we started doing research we discovered NELA, the New England Leather Alliance puts on a twice-yearly "Fetish Fair Flea" (FFF) - a kind of Fetish conference. This seemed like a good place to start.

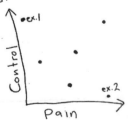

Not us!

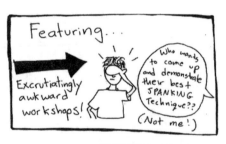

Featuring...

Excrutiatingly awkward workshops!

Who wants to come up and demonstrate their best SPANKING Technique??

(Not me!)

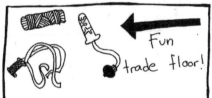

Fun trade floor!

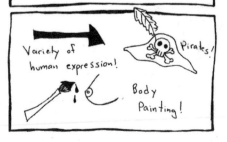

Variety of human expression!

Pirates!

Body Painting!

The FFF had two main highlights - one was a workshop lead by Japanese Fetish guru, Midori.

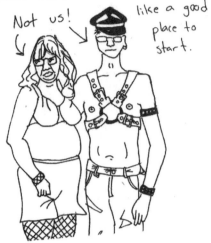

Lecture Outline
I ⁓⁓
  a ⁓⁓
  b ⁓⁓
  c ⁓⁓
II ⁓⁓

She explained a theory for locating one's interests on a kind of Fetish graph with two axes:

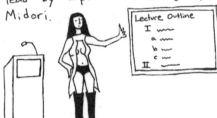

ex.1

ex.2

Control

Pain

Thus, ex.1 on the graph might enjoy activities such as:

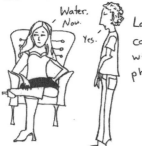

Water.
Now.
Yes.

Lots of control play with little physical pain.

Whereas ex.2 would be more like...

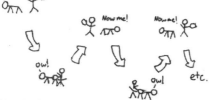

spank me!
Now me!
Now me!
ow!
ow!
etc.

Her talk was a refreshing break from all the "Dom/Sub" language.

The second highlight was a "human drumming" workshop taught by an awesome, down to earth woman (and one of the very few people of color at the conference.)
While she was in the fetish scene, she seemed less interested in pain or control, and more in interesting sensation and interaction.

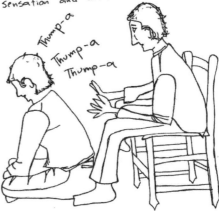

Thump-a
Thump-a
Thump-a

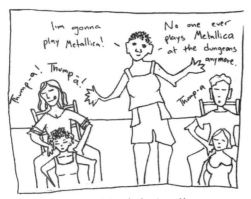

I'm gonna play Metallica!
No one ever plays Metallica at the dungeons anymore.
Thump-a!, Thump-a!
Thump-a

We later attended another drumming event (very fun) which led to our first "play party" invitation.
Our drummer friend explained that she liked to hold events around each solstice - we were all for it!

We spent a good deal of time discussing in preparation for the party, realizing we basically had no idea what we were in for.
A few very sweet party-goers answered a lot of our newbie questions.
And then, early on, we were approached very actively by a latex-clad dom.

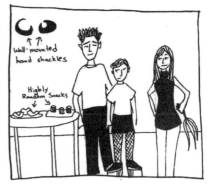

Wall-mounted hand shackles

Highly Random Snacks

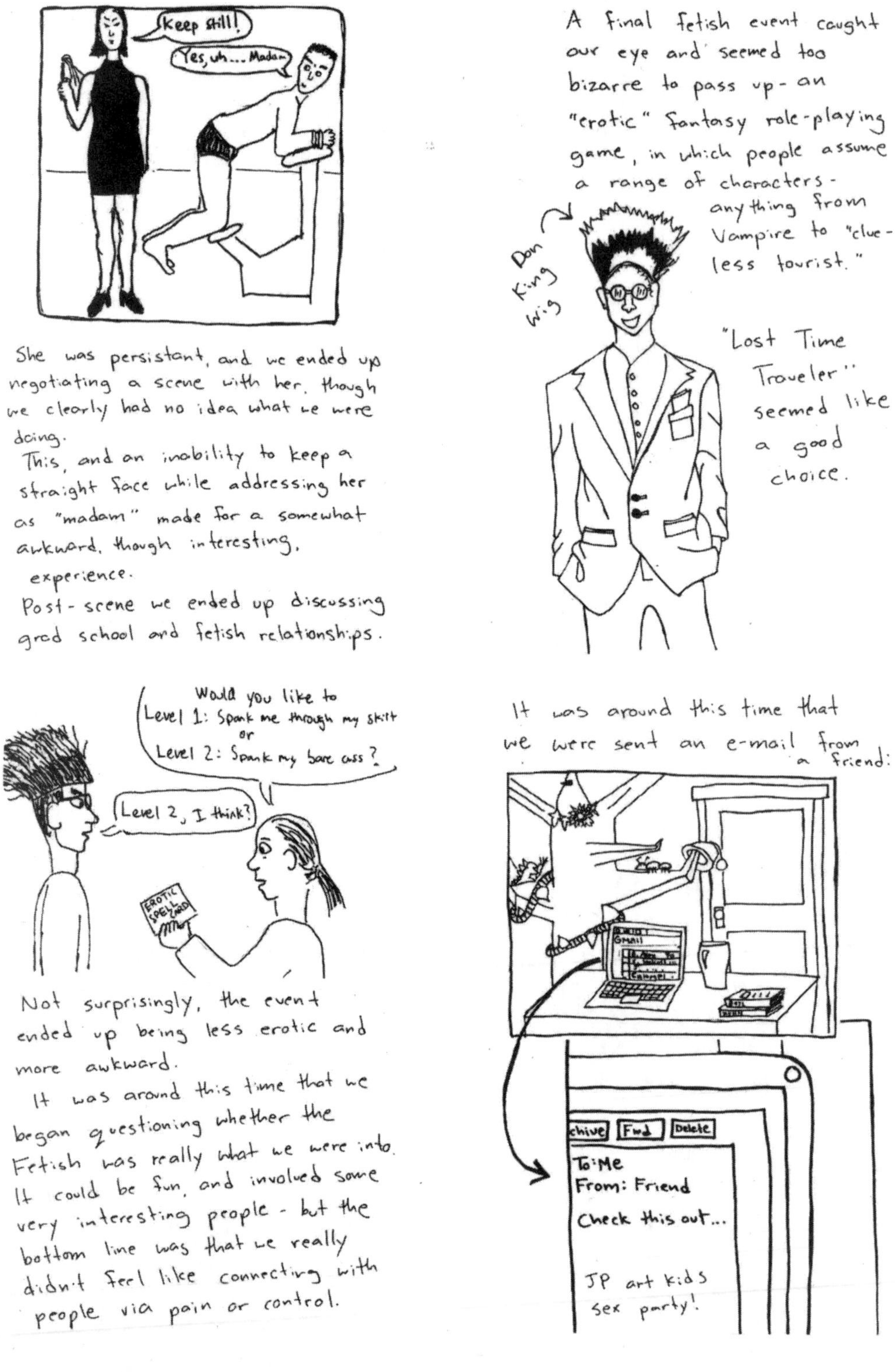
Keep still!
Yes, uh... Madam
She was persistant, and we ended up negotiating a scene with her, though we clearly had no idea what we were doing.
This, and an inability to keep a straight face while addressing her as "madam" made for a somewhat awkward, though interesting, experience.
Post-scene we ended up discussing grad school and fetish relationships.
A final fetish event caught our eye and seemed too bizarre to pass up - an "erotic" fantasy role-playing game, in which people assume a range of characters - anything from Vampire to "clue-less tourist."
Don King Wig
"Lost Time Traveler" seemed like a good choice.
Would you like to
Level 1: Spank me through my skirt
or
Level 2: Spank my bare ass?
Level 2, I think?
EROTIC SPELL CARD
Not surprisingly, the event ended up being less erotic and more awkward.
It was around this time that we began questioning whether the Fetish was really what we were into. It could be fun, and involved some very interesting people - but the bottom line was that we really didn't feel like connecting with people via pain or control.
It was around this time that we were sent an e-mail from a friend:
GMAIL
chive
Fwd
Delete
To: Me
From: Friend
Check this out...
JP art kids sex party!

The folks seeking fellow sex-partiers seemed right up our alley, proclaiming the space "feminist and queer-friendly!" Good pictures, too!

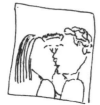

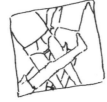

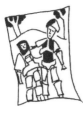

We sent a picture of ourselves dressed as robots and got an enthusiastic reply - this seemed like a good sign!

Then two years ago we switched from nonmonogamous to polyamorous. Heather is our secondary
My husband is in New Jersey with his secondary

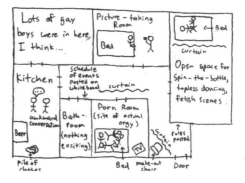

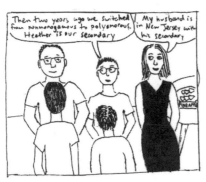

The first hour or so was surprisingly similar to an average party - milling around, eating snacks, making small talk. We ran into two girls we knew from the drummer's party and learned a little more about their situation. Simpsons references were exchanged! Things were looking up!

An official invite was extended. This would be our first non-Fetish sex party! Once again much was discussed - boundaries, ground-rules, what to wear?? Once again, we had very little idea what to expect. Upon arrival we found:

Lots of gay boys were in here, I think...
Picture-taking Room
Bed
Bed
curtain
Open space for Spin-the-bottle, topless dancing, Fetish scenes.
Kitchen
Schedule of events posted on whiteboard
curtain
awkward conversation
Beer
Bath-room (nothing exciting)
Porn Room (site of actual orgy)
TV
Curtain
rules posted
Pile of clothes
Bed
make-out chair
Door

Things continued to progress with... Naked Dancing!

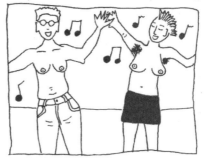

Spin the Bottle!

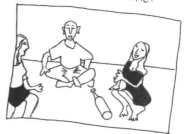

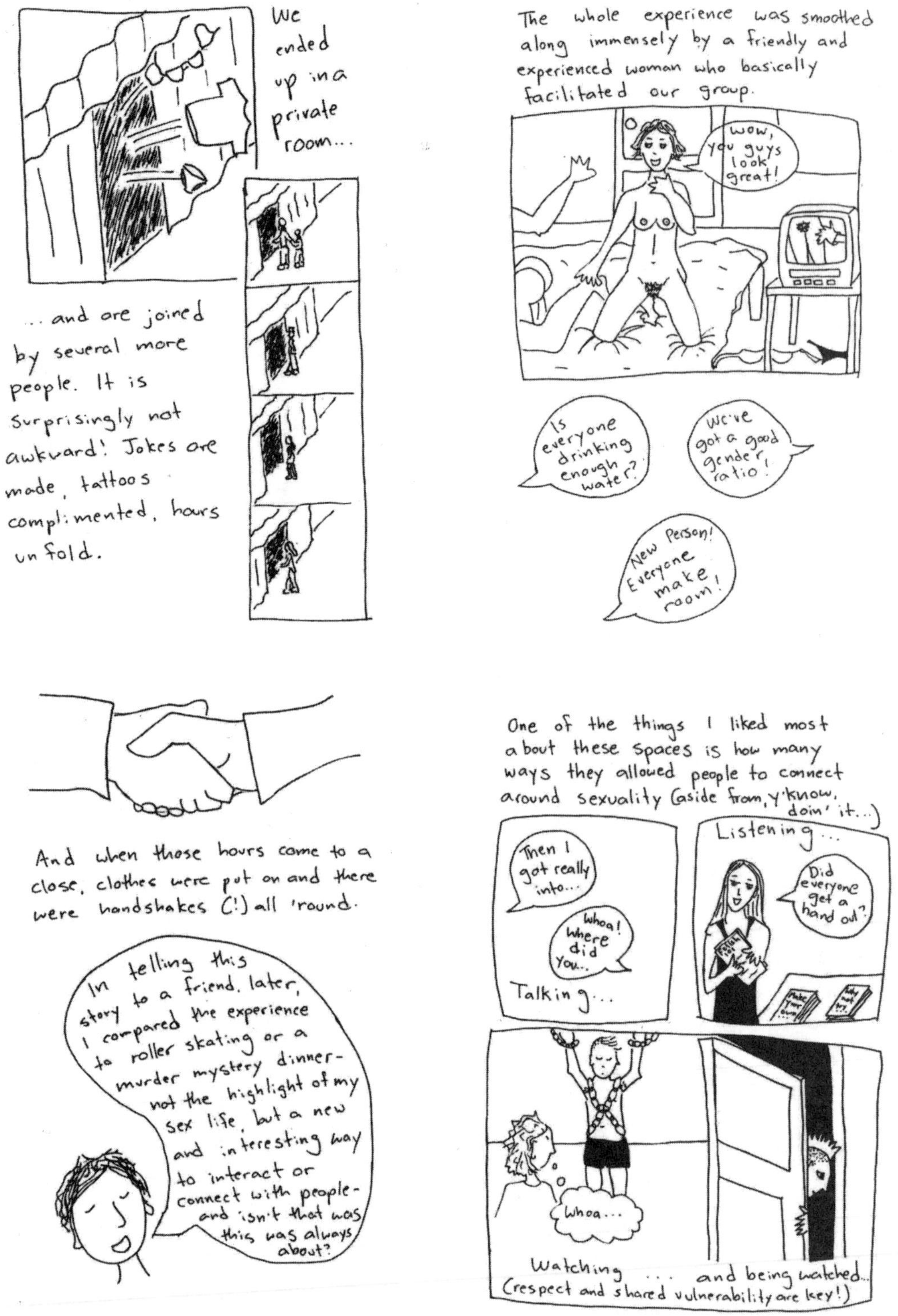
We ended up in a private room...
... and are joined by several more people. It is surprisingly not awkward! Jokes are made, tattoos complimented, hours unfold.
The whole experience was smoothed along immensely by a friendly and experienced woman who basically facilitated our group.
wow, you guys look great!
Is everyone drinking enough water?
We've got a good gender ratio!
New Person! Everyone make room!
And when those hours come to a close, clothes were put on and there were handshakes (!) all 'round.
In telling this story to a friend, later, I compared the experience to roller skating or a murder mystery dinner- not the highlight of my sex life, but a new and interesting way to interact or connect with people- and isn't that was this was always about?
One of the things I liked most about these spaces is how many ways they allowed people to connect around sexuality (aside from, y'know, doin' it...)
Then I got really into...
Whoa! Where did you...
Talking...
Listening...
Did everyone get a hand out?
Whoa...
Watching ... and being watched...
(respect and shared vulnerability are key!)

And, of course, new and interesting social ground continues to be broken as new friends turn up in unlikely places...
25¢
25¢
25¢
25¢
25¢
Hmm I know that guy from somewhere, but where? Not work or - ohhhhhh ......

Addendum: I ♡ my doctor
You want to get tested again? Are you still with the same partner?
Well... yeah but... XXX... XXX... XXX...
Totally embarrassed
OK well, sounds like you're fine but we'll do some standard tests.
Not an eyelash batted!

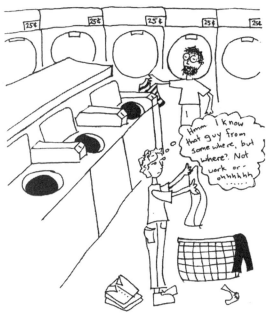

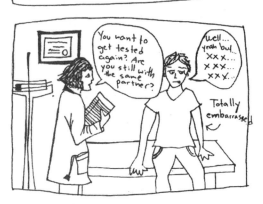

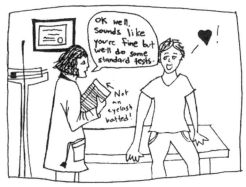

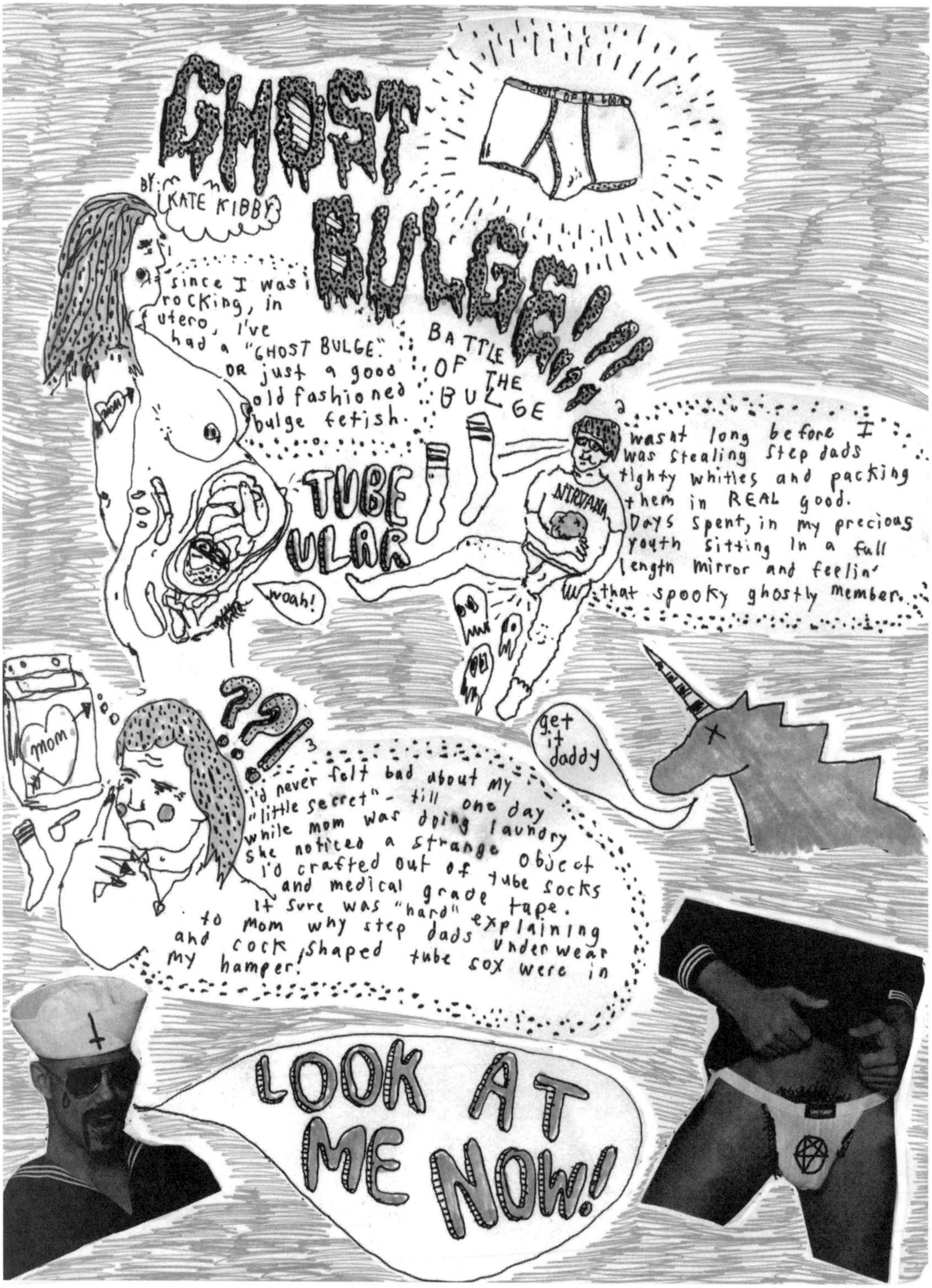
GHOST BULGE!!!
BY: KATE KIBBY
since I was i rocking, in utero, I've had a "GHOST BULGE" OR just a good old fashioned bulge fetish.
BATTLE OF THE BULGE
TUBE ULAR
woah!
wasn't long before I was stealing step dads tighty whities and packing them in REAL good. Days spent, in my precious youth sitting in a full length mirror and feelin' that spooky ghostly member.
NIRVANA
mom
??!
get it daddy
i'd never felt bad about my "little secret" - till one day while mom was doing laundry she noticed a strange object i'd crafted out of tube socks and medical grade tape. It sure was "hard" explaining to mom why step dads underwear and cock shaped tube sox were in my hamper!
LOOK AT ME NOW!

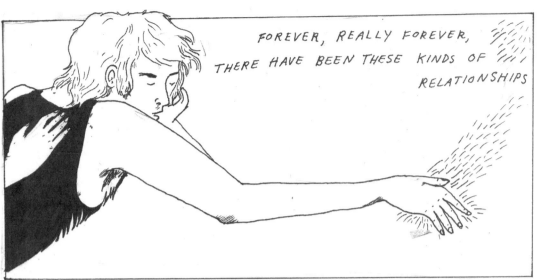

FOREVER, REALLY FOREVER, THERE HAVE BEEN THESE KINDS OF RELATIONSHIPS

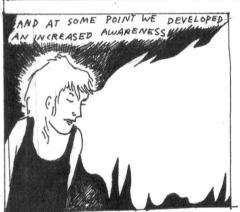

AND AT SOME POINT WE DEVELOPED AN INCREASED AWARENESS

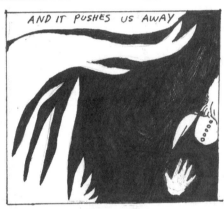

AND IT PUSHES US AWAY

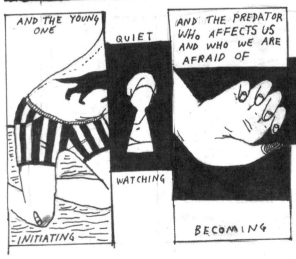

AND THE YOUNG ONE

QUIET

WATCHING

INITIATING

AND THE PREDATOR WHO AFFECTS US AND WHO WE ARE AFRAID OF

BECOMING

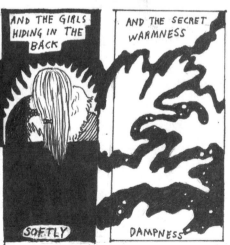

AND THE GIRLS HIDING IN THE BACK

SOFTLY

AND THE SECRET WARMNESS

DAMPNESS

AND MENTORS
AND DEMONS
I READ THE HALLOWEEN TREE BY RAY BRADBURY AND
IT FILLS ME WITH THIS PERSONAL LONGING FOR A PRE-TEEN BOY-NESS
AHHHH
ROOOOO
I FEEL THAT WAY BUT I AM ALSO AN ADULT
HE SAYS
I FEEL THAT WAY ALSO BUT WHY IS IT MALE
SHE SAYS
MY FRIENDS ARE OF A WIDE SPECTRUM
1977
1992
8
1988
2010
WE TRY TO MAKE SENSE OF THESE DESTRUCTIVE STRUCTURES
WE ATTEMPT TO REGAIN WHAT WE HAVE LOST
I ASK QUESTIONS LIKE
CAN THERE EVER BE A CONSENSUALLY & SENSUALLY UNBALANCED POWER DYNAMIC AND IS 18 AN ARBITRARY NUMBER AND IS TIME REAL AND EXPERIENCES ARE AND WHY DO YOU WANT TO SLEEP WITH SOMEONE TEN YEARS YOUNGER THAN YOU AND WHO AM I TO VILLIFY ANYONE'S SEX AND WHERE DOES MY CRITICISM OF BULL SHIT LEGALITY END AND WHEN DO WE INADVERTANTLY ENDORSE IT AND WHAT IS APPROPRIATENESS AND AND AND
WILL I EVER BE A SOFT AND WIRY NELLY FAG
& WHERE ARE OUR
ELDER QUEERS
DEAD BEFORE THEIR TIME
I WANT TO SIT IN THE GARDEN
I WANT TO PICK UP THE FIGHT
BRICK.
WITH THESE POTENTIAL
LOVERS
PARENTS
MENTORS
DEMONS
PREDATORS
COMRADES
FRIENDS
GONE TO THE NEXT REALM
LEAVING US TO RE-INVENT AND DRAW INCOHERENTLY

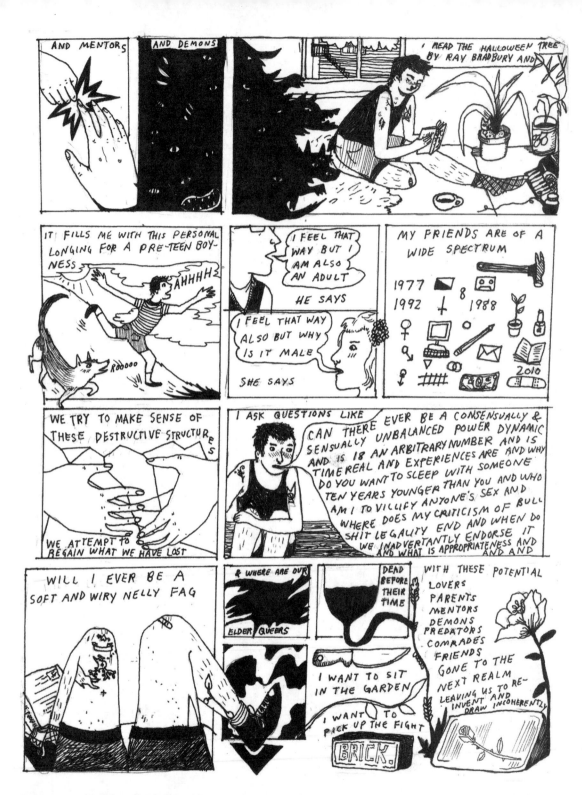

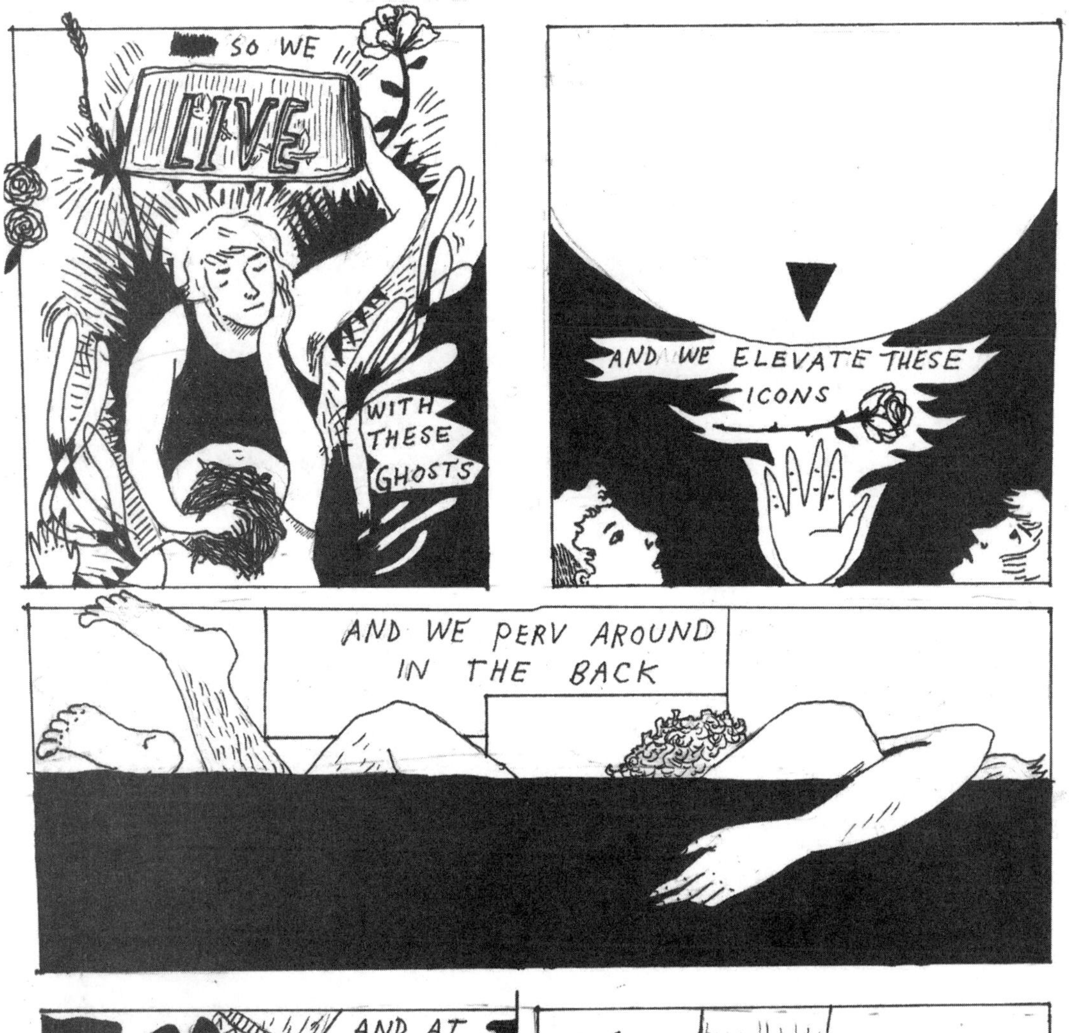
[redacted] SO WE
LIVE
WITH THESE GHOSTS
AND WE ELEVATE THESE ICONS
AND WE PERV AROUND IN THE BACK
AND AT VARIABLE LEVELS OF OKAY-NESS,
WE WALK THESE BOUNDARIES.

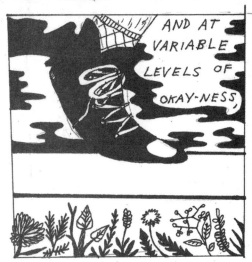

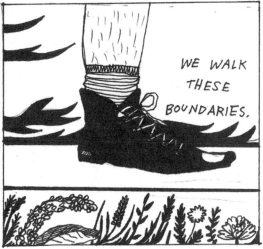

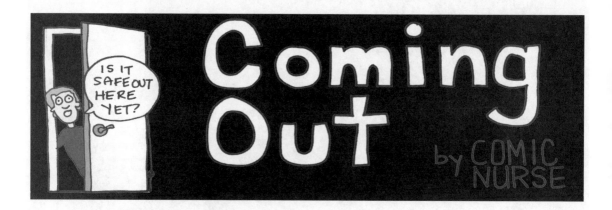

Coming Out by COMIC NURSE

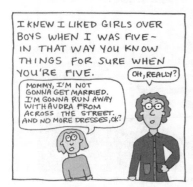

I KNEW I LIKED GIRLS OVER BOYS WHEN I WAS FIVE — IN THAT WAY YOU KNOW THINGS FOR SURE WHEN YOU'RE FIVE.

MOMMY, I'M NOT GONNA GET MARRIED. I'M GONNA RUN AWAY WITH AUDRA FROM ACROSS THE STREET, AND NO MORE DRESSES, OK?

OH, REALLY?

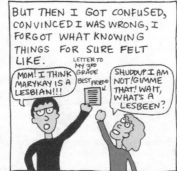

BUT THEN I GOT CONFUSED, CONVINCED I WAS WRONG, I FORGOT WHAT KNOWING THINGS FOR SURE FELT LIKE.

MOM! I THINK MARYKAY IS A LESBIAN!!!

LETTER TO MY 3RD GRADE BEST FRIEND

SHUDDUP I AM NOT! GIMME THAT! WAIT, WHAT'S A LESBEEN?

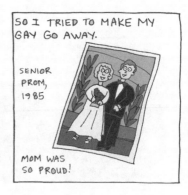

SO I TRIED TO MAKE MY GAY GO AWAY.

SENIOR PROM, 1985

MOM WAS SO PROUD!

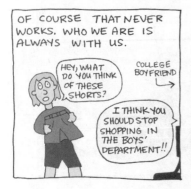

OF COURSE THAT NEVER WORKS. WHO WE ARE IS ALWAYS WITH US.

HEY, WHAT DO YOU THINK OF THESE SHORTS?

COLLEGE BOYFRIEND →

I THINK YOU SHOULD STOP SHOPPING IN THE BOYS' DEPARTMENT!!

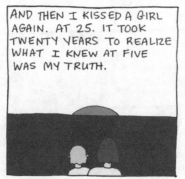

AND THEN I KISSED A GIRL AGAIN. AT 25. IT TOOK TWENTY YEARS TO REALIZE WHAT I KNEW AT FIVE WAS MY TRUTH.

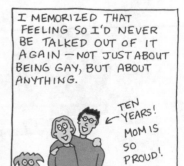

I MEMORIZED THAT FEELING SO I'D NEVER BE TALKED OUT OF IT AGAIN — NOT JUST ABOUT BEING GAY, BUT ABOUT ANYTHING.

TEN YEARS! MOM IS SO PROUD!

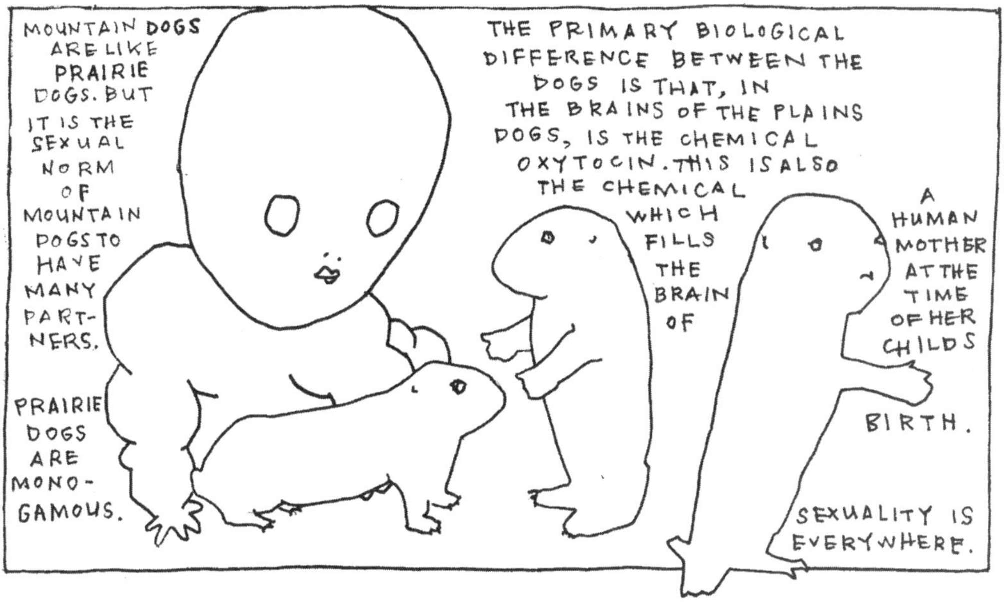
MOUNTAIN DOGS ARE LIKE PRAIRIE DOGS. BUT IT IS THE SEXUAL NORM OF MOUNTAIN DOGS TO HAVE MANY PART- NERS.
PRAIRIE DOGS ARE MONO- GAMOUS.
THE PRIMARY BIOLOGICAL DIFFERENCE BETWEEN THE DOGS IS THAT, IN THE BRAINS OF THE PLAINS DOGS, IS THE CHEMICAL OXYTOCIN. THIS IS ALSO THE CHEMICAL WHICH FILLS THE BRAIN OF
A HUMAN MOTHER AT THE TIME OF HER CHILDS BIRTH.
SEXUALITY IS EVERYWHERE.

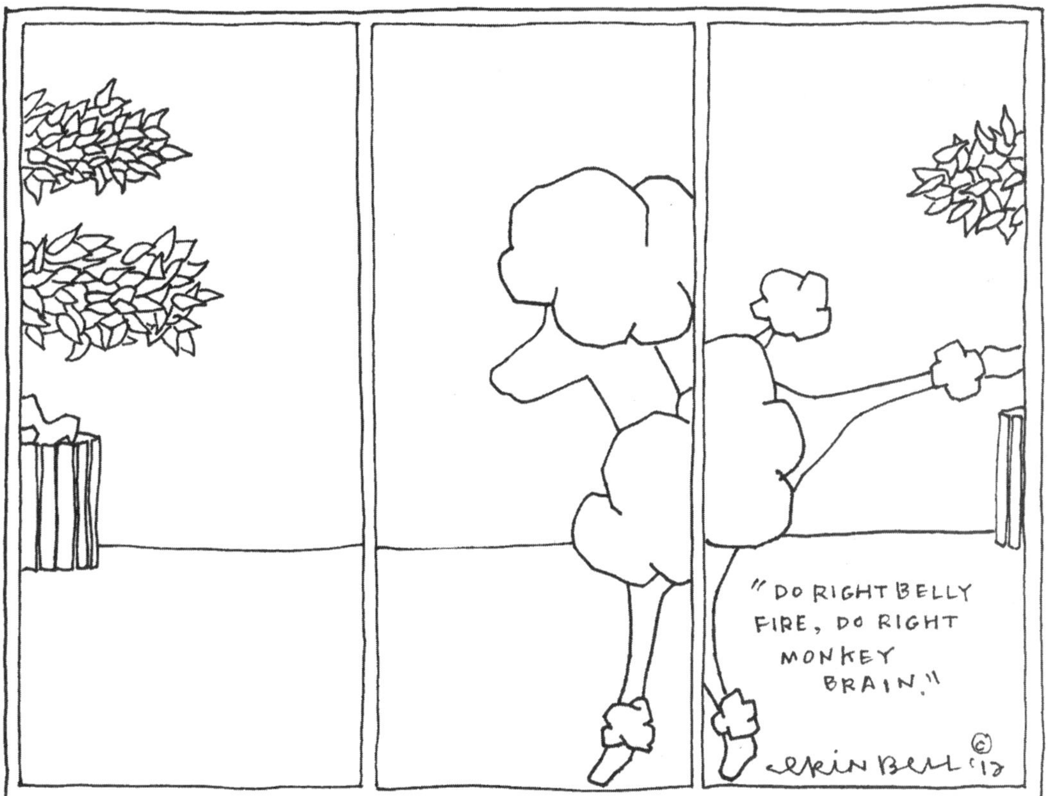
"DO RIGHT BELLY FIRE, DO RIGHT MONKEY BRAIN."
ERIN BELL ©'12

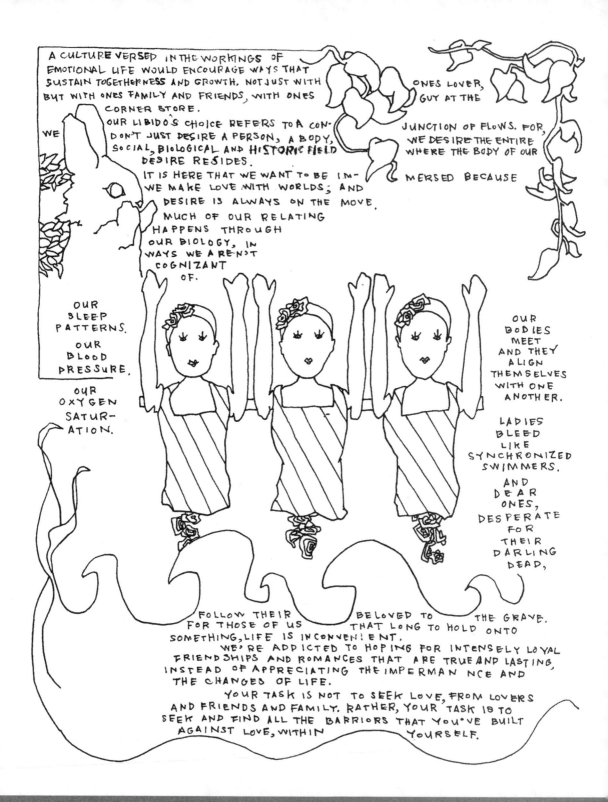

A CULTURE VERSED IN THE WORKINGS OF EMOTIONAL LIFE WOULD ENCOURAGE WAYS THAT SUSTAIN TOGETHERNESS AND GROWTH, NOT JUST WITH ONES LOVER, GUY AT THE BUT WITH ONES FAMILY AND FRIENDS, WITH ONES CORNER STORE.

WE OUR LIBIDO'S CHOICE REFERS TO A CON- DON'T JUST DESIRE A PERSON, A BODY, SOCIAL, BIOLOGICAL AND HISTORIC FIELD DESIRE RESIDES. JUNCTION OF FLOWS. FOR, WE DESIRE THE ENTIRE WHERE THE BODY OF OUR

IT IS HERE THAT WE WANT TO BE IM- WE MAKE LOVE WITH WORLDS; AND DESIRE IS ALWAYS ON THE MOVE. MERSED BECAUSE MUCH OF OUR RELATING HAPPENS THROUGH OUR BIOLOGY, IN WAYS WE AREN'T COGNIZANT OF.

OUR SLEEP PATTERNS. OUR BLOOD PRESSURE.

OUR OXYGEN SATUR- ATION.

OUR BODIES MEET AND THEY ALIGN THEMSELVES WITH ONE ANOTHER.

LADIES BLEED LIKE SYNCHRONIZED SWIMMERS. AND DEAR ONES, DESPERATE FOR THEIR DARLING DEAD,

FOLLOW THEIR BELOVED TO THE GRAVE. FOR THOSE OF US THAT LONG TO HOLD ONTO SOMETHING, LIFE IS INCONVENIENT. WE'RE ADDICTED TO HOPING FOR INTENSELY LOYAL FRIENDSHIPS AND ROMANCES THAT ARE TRUE AND LASTING, INSTEAD OF APPRECIATING THE IMPERMANCE AND THE CHANGES OF LIFE.

YOUR TASK IS NOT TO SEEK LOVE, FROM LOVERS AND FRIENDS AND FAMILY. RATHER, YOUR TASK IS TO SEEK AND FIND ALL THE BARRIORS THAT YOU'VE BUILT AGAINST LOVE, WITHIN YOURSELF.

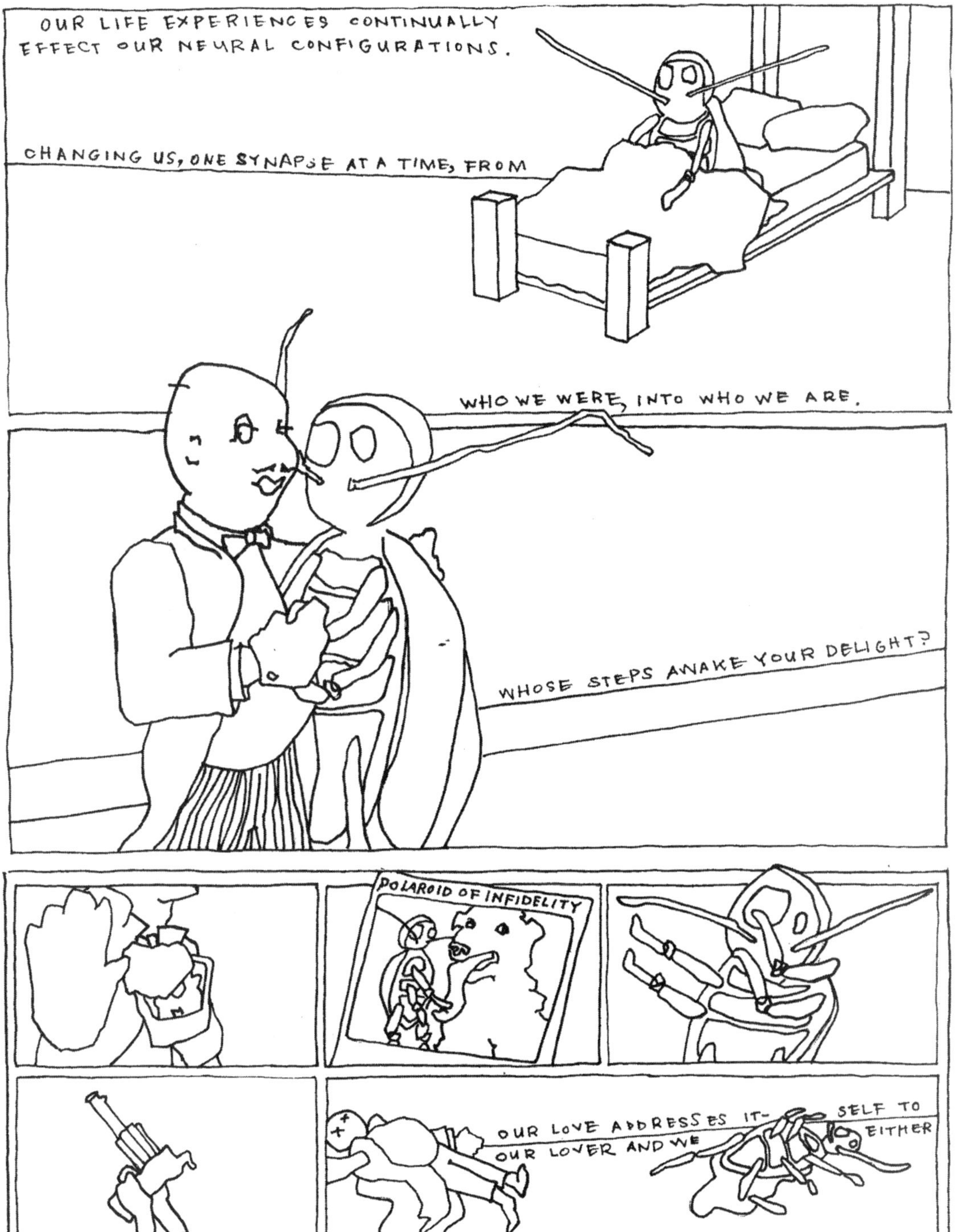
OUR LIFE EXPERIENCES CONTINUALLY EFFECT OUR NEURAL CONFIGURATIONS.
CHANGING US, ONE SYNAPSE AT A TIME, FROM
WHO WE WERE, INTO WHO WE ARE.
WHOSE STEPS AWAKE YOUR DELIGHT?
POLAROID OF INFIDELITY
OUR LOVE ADDRESSES IT- SELF TO
OUR LOVER AND WE EITHER
OPEN MORE SPACIOUS TERRITORIES, OR WE CLOSE ONE ANOTHER OFF.

WHAT'S IN YOUR MIND'S
EYE WHEN YOU ARE IN THE
THROWS OF ECSTASY?   IF WE AREN'T PERPET-
UALLY ELECTRIC WITH OUR LOVER WE FEEL WE
ARE MISSING OUT ON THE PINNACLE OF
RELATEDNESS.
FOR THOSE
CONCERNED FOR
THE GROWTH OF
ANOTHER,
THEY FOSTER
THAT GROWTH
THROUGH
CONSISTENCY.
THE FIRST ORGAN
TO SUFFER
PRIVITIZATION
IN THE

VICTORIAN
WHITE-WASHING
OF BODIES
WAS THE
ANUS.
DESIRE
AND
SEXUALITY
ARE CAPABLE
OF
CALLING
INTO
QUESTION
THE
ESTABLISHED
ORDER
OF
SOCIETY.

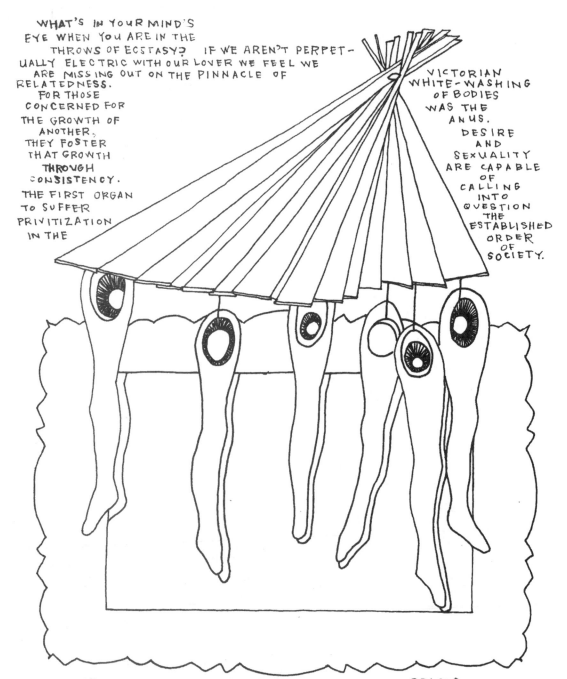

SEXUALITY AND LOVE DREAM OF WIDE OPEN SPACES.
THE VOYAGE OF DISCOVERY
CONSISTS, NOT IN SEEKING NEW LANDSCAPES,
BUT IN HAVING NEW EYES.

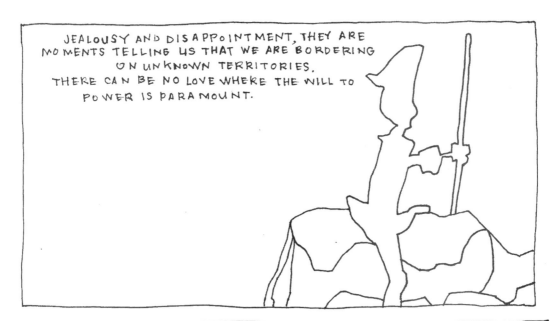

JEALOUSY AND DISAPPOINTMENT, THEY ARE MOMENTS TELLING US THAT WE ARE BORDERING ON UNKNOWN TERRITORIES.
THERE CAN BE NO LOVE WHERE THE WILL TO POWER IS PARAMOUNT.

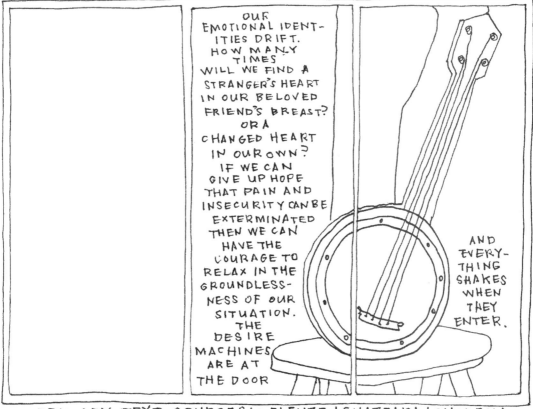

OUR EMOTIONAL IDENTITIES DRIFT. HOW MANY TIMES WILL WE FIND A STRANGER'S HEART IN OUR BELOVED FRIEND'S BREAST? OR A CHANGED HEART IN OUR OWN? IF WE CAN GIVE UP HOPE THAT PAIN AND INSECURITY CAN BE EXTERMINATED THEN WE CAN HAVE THE COURAGE TO RELAX IN THE GROUNDLESSNESS OF OUR SITUATION. THE DESIRE MACHINES ARE AT THE DOOR

AND EVERYTHING SHAKES WHEN THEY ENTER.

— PRIMARY TEXT SOURCES: DELEUZE + GUATTARI + CHODRON —

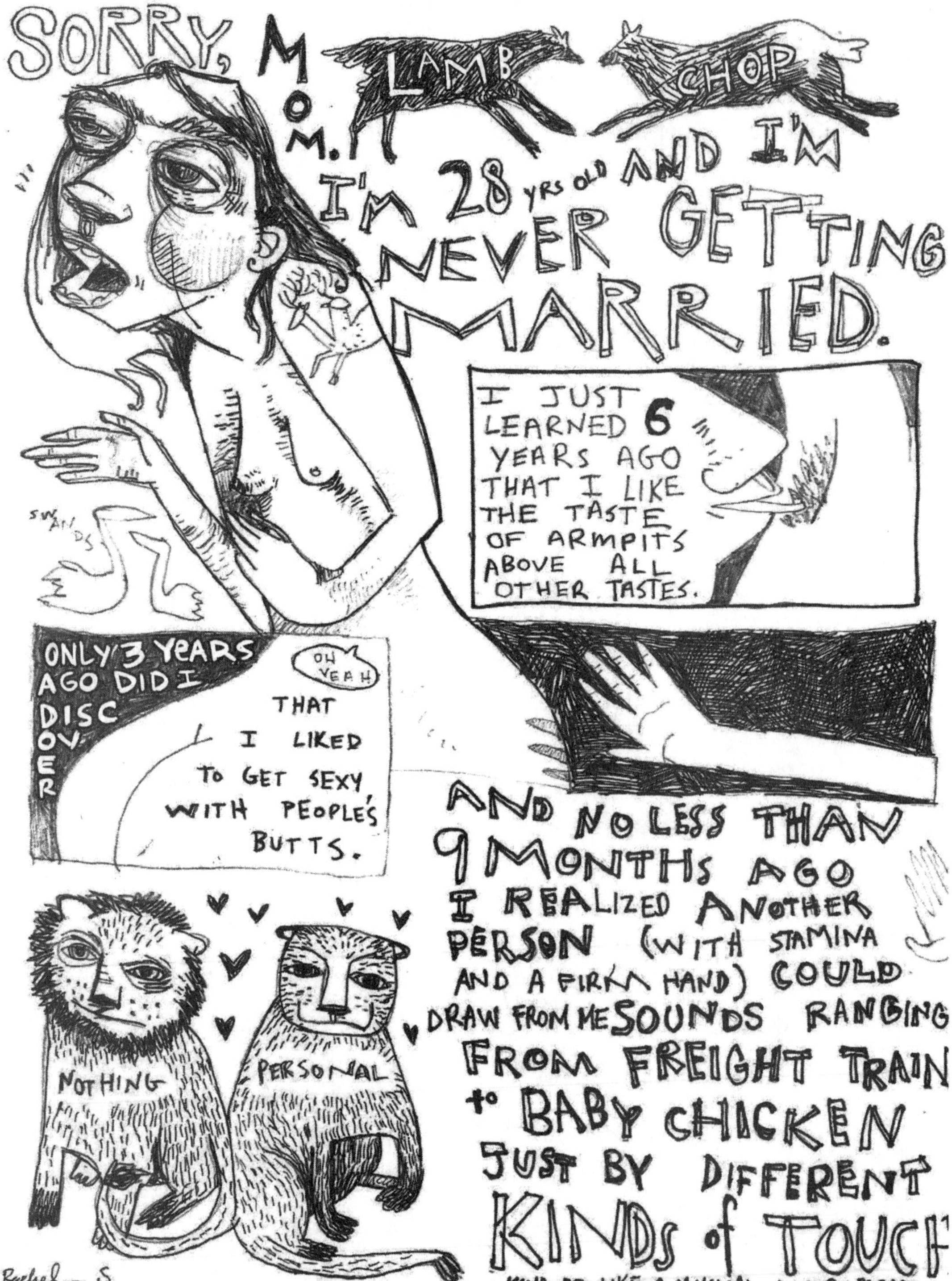
SORRY, MOM.
LAMB
CHOP
I'M 28 YRS OLD AND I'M NEVER GETTING MARRIED.
I JUST LEARNED 6 YEARS AGO THAT I LIKE THE TASTE OF ARMPITS ABOVE ALL OTHER TASTES.
SWANDS
ONLY 3 YEARS AGO DID I DISCOVER
OH YEAH
THAT I LIKED TO GET SEXY WITH PEOPLE'S BUTTS.
AND NO LESS THAN 9 MONTHS AGO I REALIZED ANOTHER PERSON (WITH STAMINA AND A FIRM HAND) COULD DRAW FROM ME SOUNDS RANGING FROM FREIGHT TRAIN to BABY CHICKEN JUST BY DIFFERENT KINDS of TOUCH
KIND OF LIKE A MUSICAL INSTRUMENT
NOTHING
PERSONAL
Rachel S

CHAPTER FIVE:

AGE

SAIYA

My early attempts at adulthood were clumsy, before I realized that age mattered less than knowing what I felt ready for. Symbolic rites of passage such as sex and partying were done too early, in a hopeful attempt to seem more grown-up. Do the boundaries we form for ourselves always occur as a result of certain things happening before we are ready? What does it mean to grow up, to age gracefully, even as a young person?

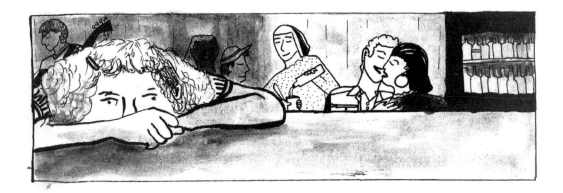

LIZA

I was born in the summer of 1986. Now, I am in my mid-twenties. Age plays a major role in my sexual health. There was a time, as one comic contributor put it, when nearly everything was a "first," but now with each new year I have fewer new sexual encounters. The people I do have sex with are the same friends I have been having sex with for years. We will never go on a date, but if we are in the same city on the right night, we will fuck. As we age, our sex retains the same pattern.

SAIYA

As a kid, I had an aversion to the flowers on the wallpaper in my bedroom. I remember being sent to my room to take a nap every afternoon and staring at the clusters of pink roses. They were identical, spaced in diagonal rows and interrupted by smaller buds and leaves. The problem was that the insides of each rose in the cluster all faced in the same direction, toward me, and their arrangement made them look like a mean face. As soon as I was old enough I started covering them up with posters.

In middle school, the theme of the posters shifted significantly; cute animal pictures were replaced abruptly with Leonardo DiCaprio. Leo had an almost mystical power over me. His hair was glowing and polished, arching over his brow like a lion tail made of bronze. His face had a warm glow, too; even the pale blue eyes seemed warm and knowing. His leather jacket made his small shoulders appear sturdy and solid, like the arms of the leather chair that ruled over our living room. For me, though, the most interesting thing about him was that he seemed like neither man nor woman. He had womanly eyebrows and pouty lips. My big sister had recently moved out of our shared bedroom, and Leo became a sort of stand-in, an older girl who knew so much about boys and being famous. Leo became a strong female figure in my life. I looked to him for guidance.

When the movie *Titanic* came to theaters, I developed an obsession with a movie on the big screen that I had never experienced before. I went back three times to see it in the theater, and each time wondered at the scene in which Rose asks Jack to draw her like one of his French girls. This was the strangest feeling for me, to watch the Leo I knew from my wall patiently drawing a naked lady. In my young mind, it seemed I had uncovered a secret: that many different things defined a woman, and what was under the silk robe or the leather jacket mattered little.

It seemed like Leo was growing up faster than I was. I wanted to understand the nature of the intimacy that I witnessed between the characters, the grown-up type of feeling they seemed to have when they were together.

LIZA

Unfortunately, I am lonely and have been for a long time. This is difficult to admit because I also love not being in a relationship. Elementary school romance excluded, I've been in only four relationships that lasted longer than two months. I am proud not to feel like I need a constant partner. Independence was always important to me. Experimenting sexually with friends and strangers alike was exciting and satisfied me for years. Admitting loneliness is like disowning my independence, shaming my past self, and surrendering to my grandmother's notions of romantic priorities.

The majority of my friends are partnered up. Even those diehard punks and queers are settling down to domestic bliss. I've felt it coming for a while. That casual shift when "my plans" become "our plans." Road trips morph into cohabitation; cohabitation morphs into weddings. Perhaps I exaggerate after feeling so single for so long, but it is strange to watch so many who fought the mainstream end up in undeniably conventional relationships. Is that what I want, too?

SAIYA

When people ask me about my first kiss, I don't know what to tell them. The truth is, I have no idea. I strain to recall the magical moment when the clouds parted and the golden sun melted onto me. Was it at summer camp, around the fire? With a girl from my soccer team? With a friend from school? I honestly cannot remember. I think that for each of these kisses, I told myself, "Well *that* didn't count," and moved on. I kept going, kissing and kissing and having none of them count until I look back on them now. I think I was waiting for a kiss that meant something more, that moved me. I was waiting for a kiss that would summon the wind into the trees above me. Until then, other kissing did not count.

When I started having sex, I realized that virginity was not so simple either. I was intent on losing this thing. I was convinced I would transform into some kind of sexy phoenix when I did. Then I lost it, and felt unchanged. I came to believe that there is a technical definition of virginity that feels incomplete. The forewarnings of the pain, the blood on the sheets, and the entrance to the garden of sexual knowledge all feel like mythologies. Everyone has their own definition. The most popular idea of virginity, the penis-in-vagina land of no return, is only one way to look at it. When it comes to sex, there have been so many first times—with my first boyfriend, with a perfect stranger, with the first lady I ever went home with, even my first orgasm: each of these sticks out as an equally pivotal discovery, a flag marking new territory. There's so much fuss over the V-card, the boys in the lunchroom poking their stupid index fingers into the circle of their other hands. What about all of the other fun things to do in bed; do none of them count? What about the first time someone holds you and you feel safe? The first time you can talk to your partner, tell them what you want? The first time you set a boundary for yourself out loud?

LIZA

I do want romance again. I'm not looking for someone to grow old with or a forever home. Instead, I am interested in an opportunity to become familiar with another body and for them to be familiar with mine. After experiencing sex through a series of sporadic pairings spread out over ten years, that acclimation to someone else's body is a surreal idea. The thought of ending up with another loser terrifies me. My desire for affection makes me blind to their awfulness. To be fair, I do not consider myself an A+ partner either. I made many mistakes. I regret not having the opportunity to learn from them.

AS A CHILD I SPENT A LOT OF TIME ALONE
IN MY OWN HEAD
PST
HAHA
10
THIS CONTINUED A LONG TIME
SOMETIMES, EVEN WHEN I'M NOT,
I STILL FEEL ALONE.

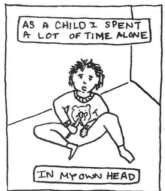

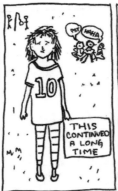

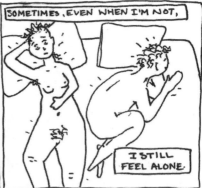

Sometimes, aging can make you feel like your life keeps repeating. In these instances, I feel less eager to write and illustrate any of my experiences. There is a lack of material with each passing year. My comics about one-night stands, STI scares, and masturbation feel recycled. I feel like I am supposed to keep living new material. Narratives too often take on a linear form that is difficult to live up to.

SAIYA

Around age fourteen I started breaking into my parents' liquor cabinet. It was a bad way to start drinking for a couple of reasons. In order to get drunk, I had to drink more than one sip, but, to keep the liquid in the bottles relatively even, I ended up drinking six different kinds of alcohol. This had a powerful effect and would make the world soften and wobble as I headed out the door for the night.

My closest friend at the time had a more serious problem. She started drinking right after school, usually a pint of cheap vodka. By the time the sun set over the trees in the park where we hung out after school, her clear bluish eyes were drooping lazily, and the bottle was almost empty. She would twist her wavy brown hair around her fingers and cackle loudly when I made fun of the boys in the park. I loved the sound of it, like a chicken squawking in the dirt. I followed her everywhere, and there was nowhere she wouldn't go. Her schemes seemed completely logical to my brave and drunken mind.

"Let's get some wine and go look at the water" was my favorite.

We would slink down the steep hill and claim a bench on the dock to look at the boats and the glowing city on the other side of the river. Sometimes I was in love with her.

At some point in the night, I felt the tide change. I started to feel that I was in over my head. Then she would say, "Let's get some whiskey and go find those guys." We trudged up the hill, the lieutenant and his weary soldier. It was always interesting to watch her find the guys and set us up. I observed her intently.

We were in the backseat of a car one afternoon, the sun still reaching through a graying sheet of clouds. We were waiting for someone, parked outside his house. I was just noticing how I could see a phantom double of the garden gnome next to the porch steps when I puked. "Oh, come on!" she said, pulling off my shirt and handing me her sweater. "I'm sorry I'm sorry," I mumbled as the car wheels screeched and we drove off. The rest of that day is flashing images, a series of pictures. We are kissing each other while the guys watch. I am following her down a staircase. She is handing me a cigarette. I am alone on the sidewalk and I don't know where she went.

My mother called her a skank, and it is true that she was the prototype of a bad influence. I needed a captain and she needed an ocean of booze. It felt natural when we kissed a boy at the same time, the three of us on the couch with our limbs twisted together, but as soon as she got bored and left the room, I had no idea what I was doing there.

I could not keep up with her and I slowly got tired of the chase. The last time I saw her, we had plans to go see a band play at a big club in the city. We got a ride there from her mom and arrived just as the doors were opening. "Let's go in!" I yelled and tried to grasp her hand as she walked toward the corner. "No, I need to get some beers first," she drawled, so we wandered down the next street to find a store. "Come on, we're gonna be late," I begged her quietly. "Relax, OK?" she snapped. She bought four beers and drank three of them by the time we made it to the show. We missed all but five minutes of the band and I sipped the last warm beer with her in the bathroom hallway.

GRAY SEX

Mat Defiler

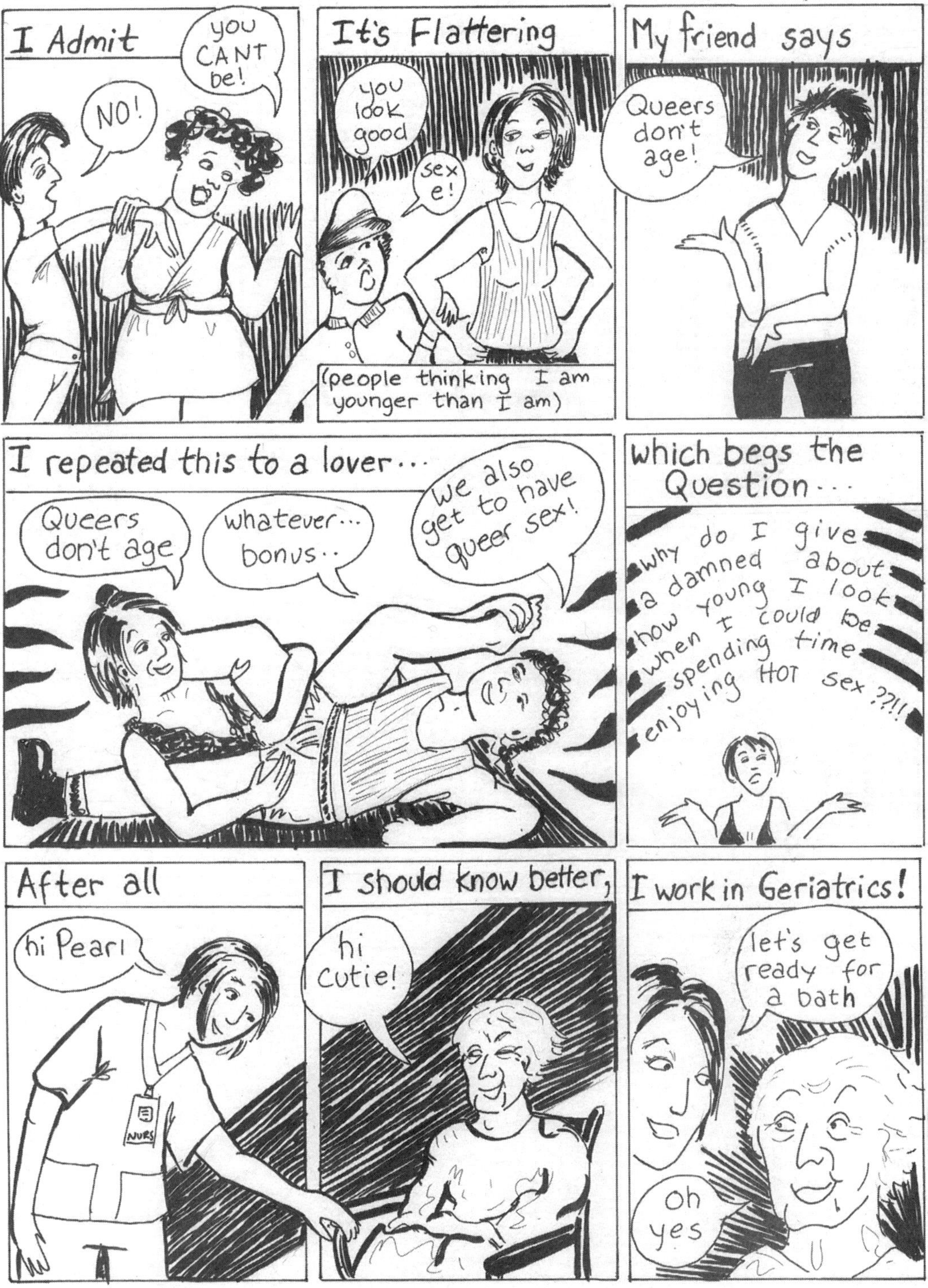
I Admit
NO!
you CANT be!
It's Flattering
you look good
sex e!
(people thinking I am younger than I am)
My friend says
Queers don't age!
I repeated this to a lover...
Queers don't age
whatever... bonus..
we also get to have queer sex!
which begs the Question...
why do I give a damned about how young I look when I could be spending time enjoying HOT sex??!!
After all
hi Pearl
NURS
I should know better,
hi Cutie!
I work in Geriatrics!
let's get ready for a bath
Oh yes

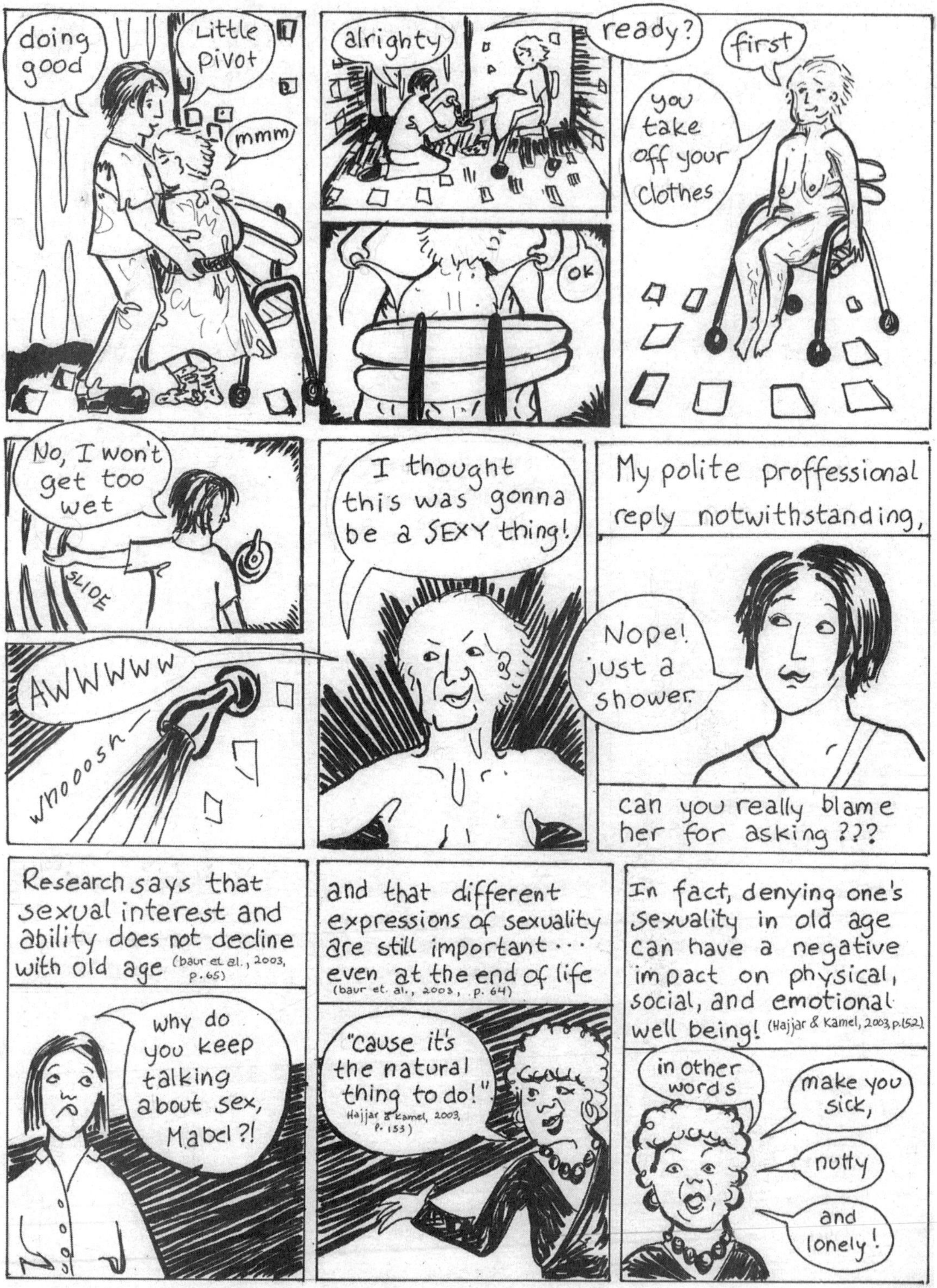

doing good
Little pivot
mmm
alrighty
ready?
OK
first
you take off your clothes
No, I won't get too wet
SLIDE
AWWWWW
whooosh
I thought this was gonna be a SEXY thing!
My polite proffessional reply notwithstanding,
Nope! just a shower.
can you really blame her for asking???
Research says that sexual interest and ability does not decline with old age (baur et al., 2003, p. 65)
why do you keep talking about sex, Mabel?!
and that different expressions of sexuality are still important... even at the end of life (baur et. al., 2003, p. 64)
"cause it's the natural thing to do!" Hajjar & Kamel, 2003, p. 153)
In fact, denying one's Sexuality in old age can have a negative impact on physical, social, and emotional well being! (Hajjar & Kamel, 2003, p. 152)
in other words
make you sick,
nutty
and lonely!

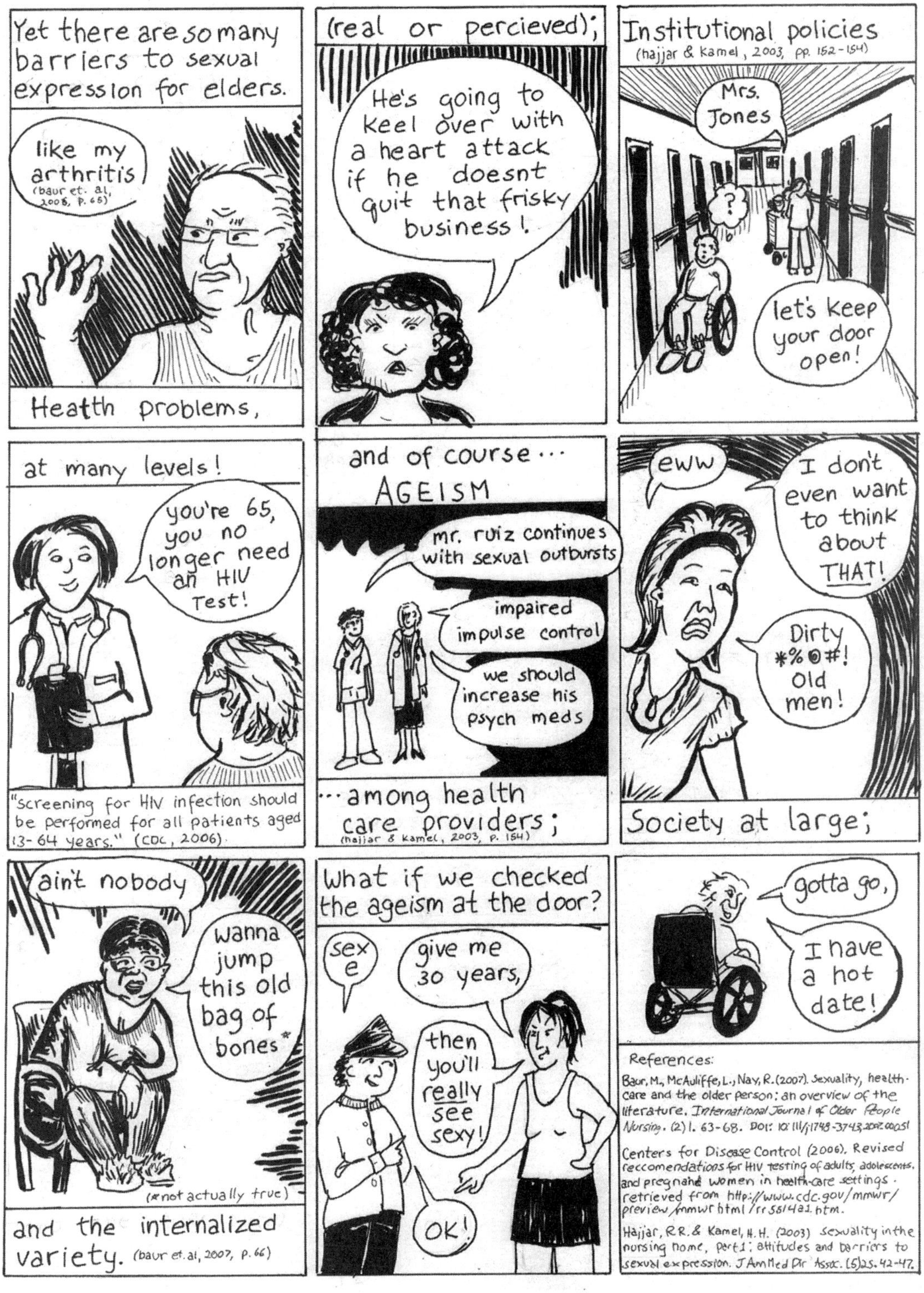
Yet there are so many barriers to sexual expression for elders.
like my arthritis
(baur et. al, 2008, p. 65)
Heatth problems,
(real or percieved);
He's going to keel over with a heart attack if he doesnt quit that frisky business!
Institutional policies
(hajjar & Kamel, 2003, pp. 152-154)
Mrs. Jones
?
let's keep your door open!
at many levels!
you're 65, you no longer need an HIV Test!
"screening for HIV infection should be performed for all patients aged 13-64 years." (CDC, 2006)
and of course...
AGEISM
mr. ruiz continues with sexual outbursts
impaired impulse control
we should increase his psych meds
...among health care providers;
(hajjar & kamel, 2003, p. 154)
eww
I don't even want to think about THAT!
Dirty *%@#! old men!
Society at large;
ain't nobody
wanna jump this old bag of bones*
(*not actually true)
and the internalized variety. (baur et. al, 2007, p. 66)
What if we checked the ageism at the door?
sex e
give me 30 years,
then you'll really see sexy!
OK!
gotta go,
I have a hot date!
References:
Baur, M., McAuliffe, L., Nay, R. (2007). Sexuality, health-care and the older person: an overview of the literature. International Journal of Older People Nursing. (2)1. 63-68. DOI: 10.111/j.1748-3743.2007.00051
Centers for Disease Control (2006). Revised reccomendations for HIV testing of adults, adolescents, and pregnant women in health-care settings. retrieved from http://www.cdc.gov/mmwr/preview/mmwr html/rr5514a1.htm.
Hajjar, R.R. & Kamel, H.H. (2003) Sexuality in the nursing home, part 1: attitudes and barriers to sexual expression. J Am Med Dir Assoc. (5)25. 42-47.

the age thing

by Brandon

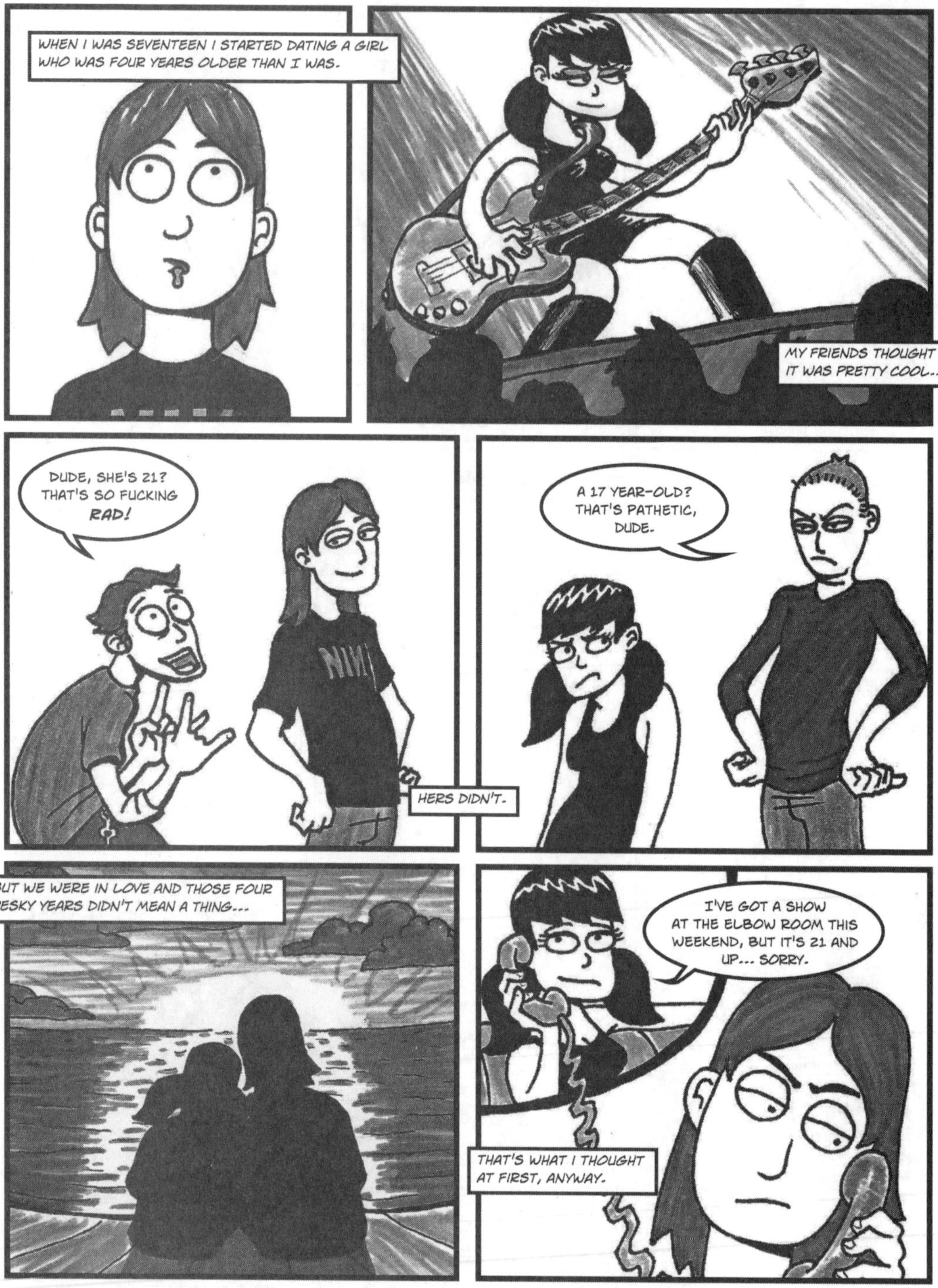
WHEN I WAS SEVENTEEN I STARTED DATING A GIRL WHO WAS FOUR YEARS OLDER THAN I WAS.
MY FRIENDS THOUGHT IT WAS PRETTY COOL...
DUDE, SHE'S 21? THAT'S SO FUCKING RAD!
HERS DIDN'T.
A 17 YEAR-OLD? THAT'S PATHETIC, DUDE.
BUT WE WERE IN LOVE AND THOSE FOUR PESKY YEARS DIDN'T MEAN A THING...
I'VE GOT A SHOW AT THE ELBOW ROOM THIS WEEKEND, BUT IT'S 21 AND UP... SORRY.
THAT'S WHAT I THOUGHT AT FIRST, ANYWAY.

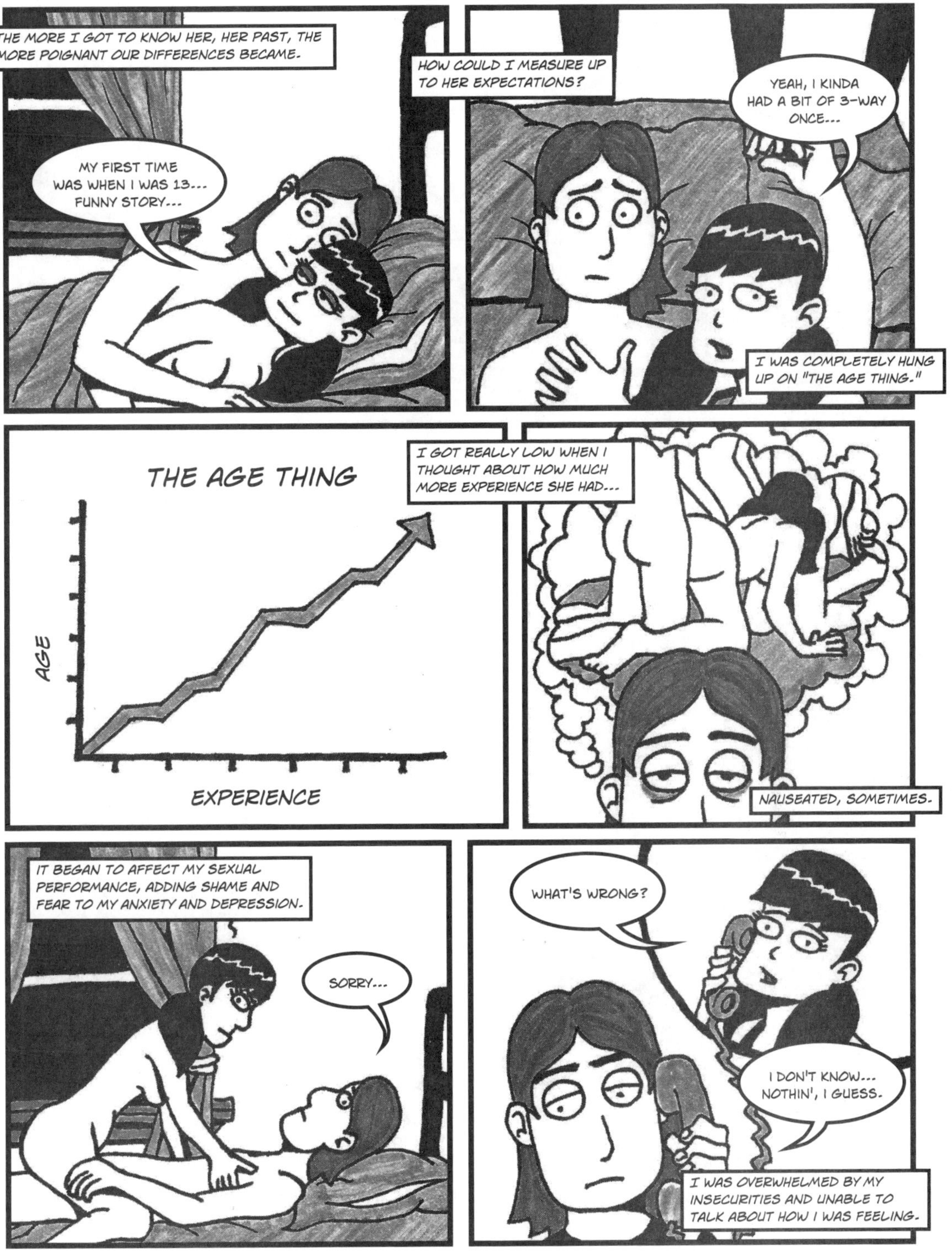
THE MORE I GOT TO KNOW HER, HER PAST, THE MORE POIGNANT OUR DIFFERENCES BECAME.
MY FIRST TIME WAS WHEN I WAS 13... FUNNY STORY...
HOW COULD I MEASURE UP TO HER EXPECTATIONS?
YEAH, I KINDA HAD A BIT OF 3-WAY ONCE...
I WAS COMPLETELY HUNG UP ON "THE AGE THING."
THE AGE THING
AGE
EXPERIENCE
I GOT REALLY LOW WHEN I THOUGHT ABOUT HOW MUCH MORE EXPERIENCE SHE HAD...
NAUSEATED, SOMETIMES.
IT BEGAN TO AFFECT MY SEXUAL PERFORMANCE, ADDING SHAME AND FEAR TO MY ANXIETY AND DEPRESSION.
SORRY...
WHAT'S WRONG?
I DON'T KNOW... NOTHIN', I GUESS.
I WAS OVERWHELMED BY MY INSECURITIES AND UNABLE TO TALK ABOUT HOW I WAS FEELING.

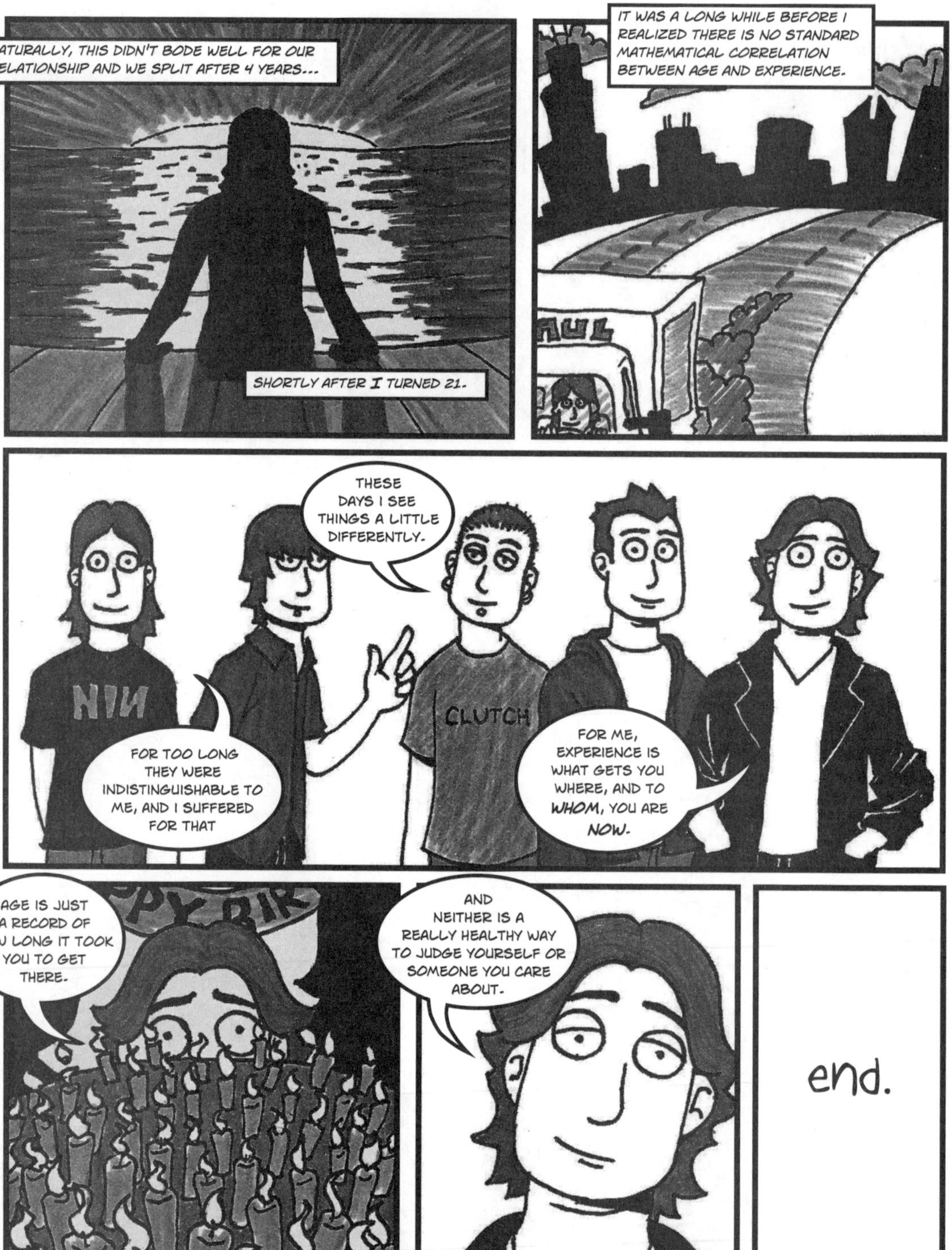
NATURALLY, THIS DIDN'T BODE WELL FOR OUR RELATIONSHIP AND WE SPLIT AFTER 4 YEARS...
SHORTLY AFTER I TURNED 21.
IT WAS A LONG WHILE BEFORE I REALIZED THERE IS NO STANDARD MATHEMATICAL CORRELATION BETWEEN AGE AND EXPERIENCE.
THESE DAYS I SEE THINGS A LITTLE DIFFERENTLY.
NIN
CLUTCH
FOR TOO LONG THEY WERE INDISTINGUISHABLE TO ME, AND I SUFFERED FOR THAT
FOR ME, EXPERIENCE IS WHAT GETS YOU WHERE, AND TO WHOM, YOU ARE NOW.
AGE IS JUST A RECORD OF HOW LONG IT TOOK YOU TO GET THERE.
AND NEITHER IS A REALLY HEALTHY WAY TO JUDGE YOURSELF OR SOMEONE YOU CARE ABOUT.
end.
© 2011

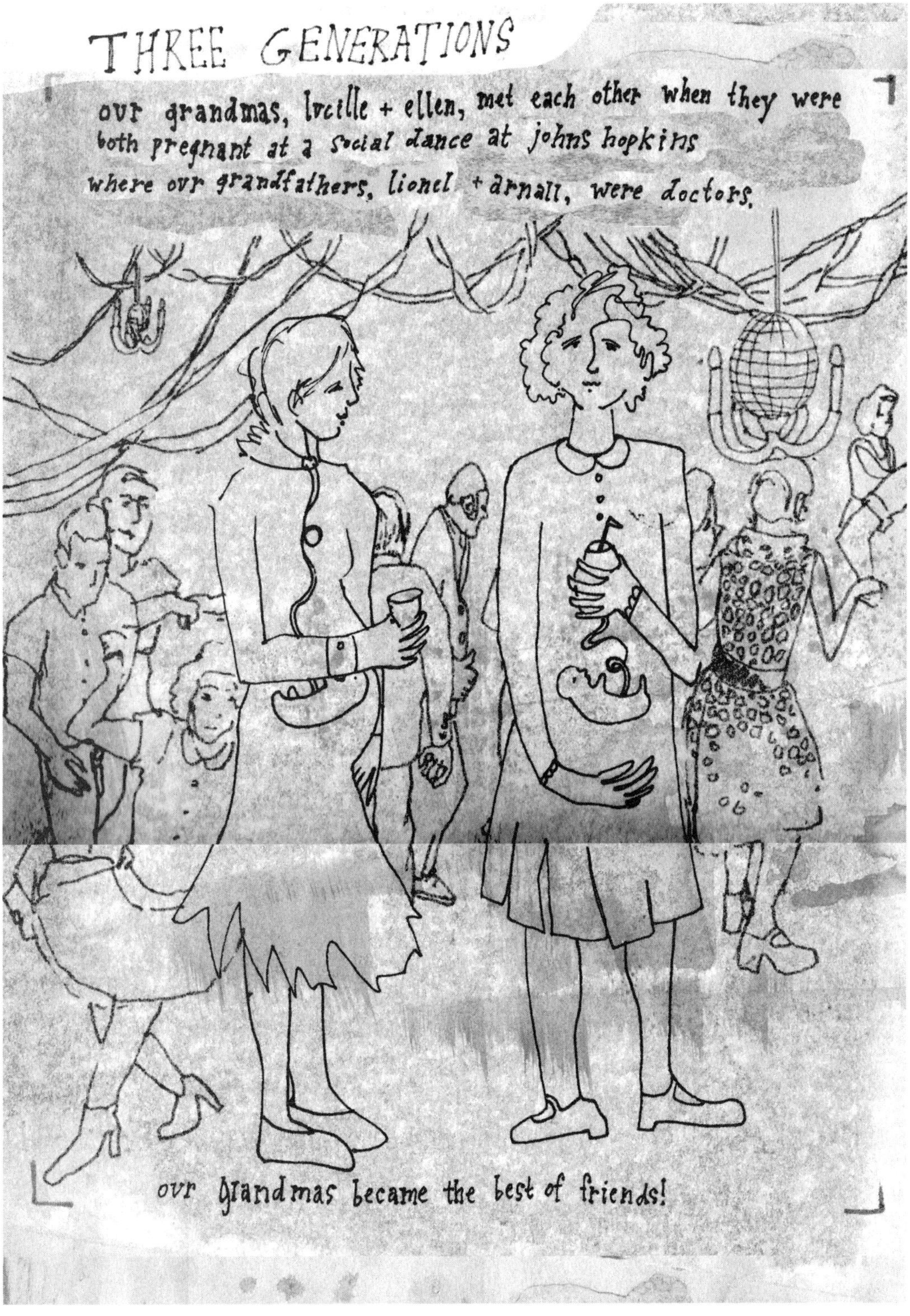
THREE GENERATIONS
our grandmas, lucille + ellen, met each other when they were both pregnant at a social dance at johns hopkins
where our grandfathers, lionel + arnall, were doctors.
our grandmas became the best of friends!

our moms, janet ruth and susan, grew up togethers. on february 8ᵗʰ, 1987 susan birthed a baby girl.

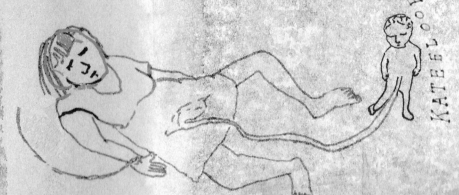

KATE BLOOD

when janet ruth heard the news, she started making a baby! 9 months later, on november 3ʳᵈ, she squirted out a baby person.

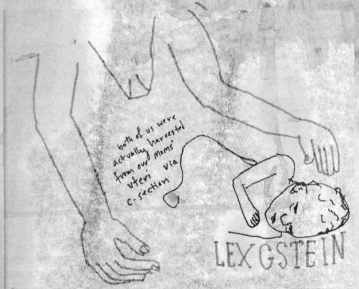

both of us were actually 'harvested' from our moms' uteri via c-section

LEX GSTEIN

and now we are sister best friends!

people ask us if we're going to synch our babies
WE ARE BOTH QUEER
maybe we'll use the same sperm donor!

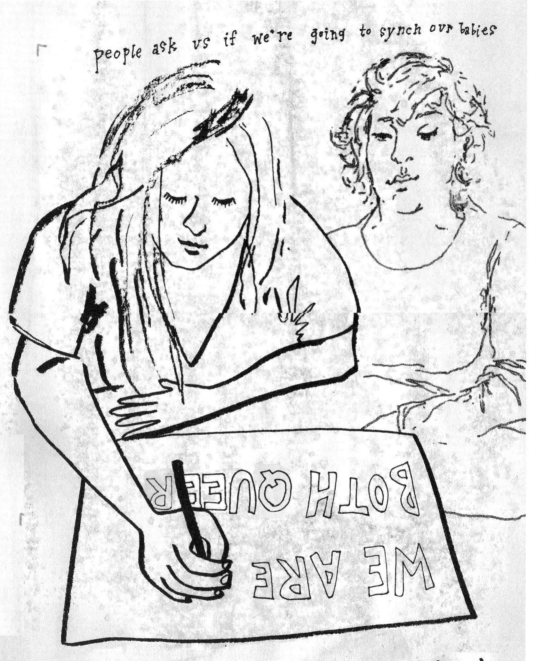

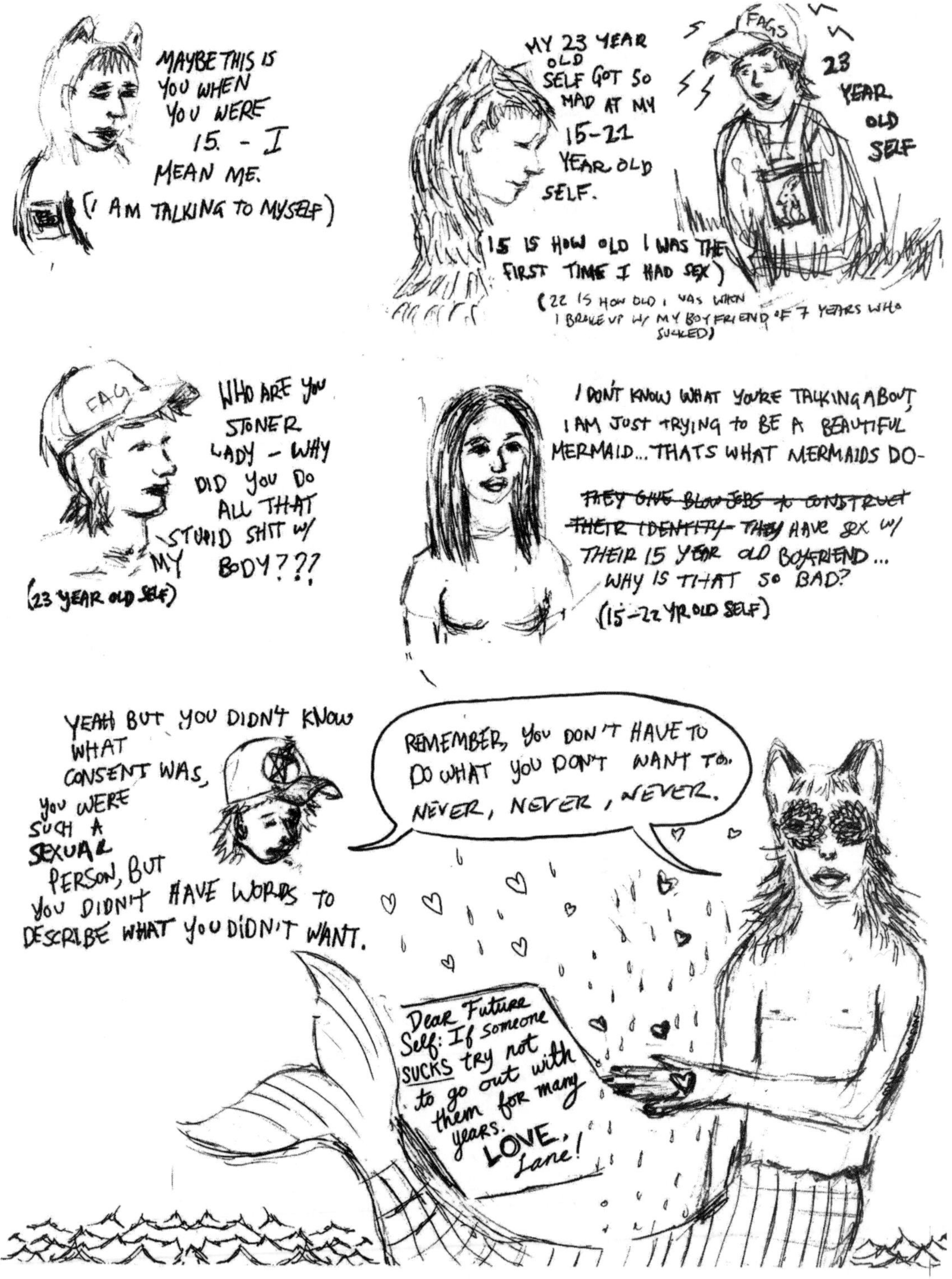
MAYBE THIS IS YOU WHEN YOU WERE 15. - I MEAN ME.
(I AM TALKING TO MYSELF)
MY 23 YEAR OLD SELF GOT SO MAD AT MY 15-21 YEAR OLD SELF.
FAGS
23 YEAR OLD SELF
(15 IS HOW OLD I WAS THE FIRST TIME I HAD SEX)
(22 IS HOW OLD I WAS WHEN I BROKE UP W/ MY BOYFRIEND OF 7 YEARS WHO SUCKED)
FAG
WHO ARE YOU STONER LADY - WHY DID YOU DO ALL THAT STUPID SHIT W/ MY BODY???
(23 YEAR OLD SELF)
I DON'T KNOW WHAT YOU'RE TALKING ABOUT, I AM JUST TRYING TO BE A BEAUTIFUL MERMAID... THATS WHAT MERMAIDS DO- ~~THEY GIVE BLOW JOBS to CONSTRUCT THEIR IDENTITY THEY~~ HAVE SEX W/ THEIR 15 YEAR OLD BOYFRIEND... WHY IS THAT SO BAD?
(15-22 YR OLD SELF)
YEAH BUT YOU DIDN'T KNOW WHAT CONSENT WAS, YOU WERE SUCH A SEXUAL PERSON, BUT YOU DIDN'T HAVE WORDS TO DESCRIBE WHAT YOU DIDN'T WANT.
REMEMBER, YOU DON'T HAVE TO DO WHAT YOU DON'T WANT TO. NEVER, NEVER, NEVER.
Dear Future Self: If someone SUCKS try not to go out with them for many years. LOVE, Lane!

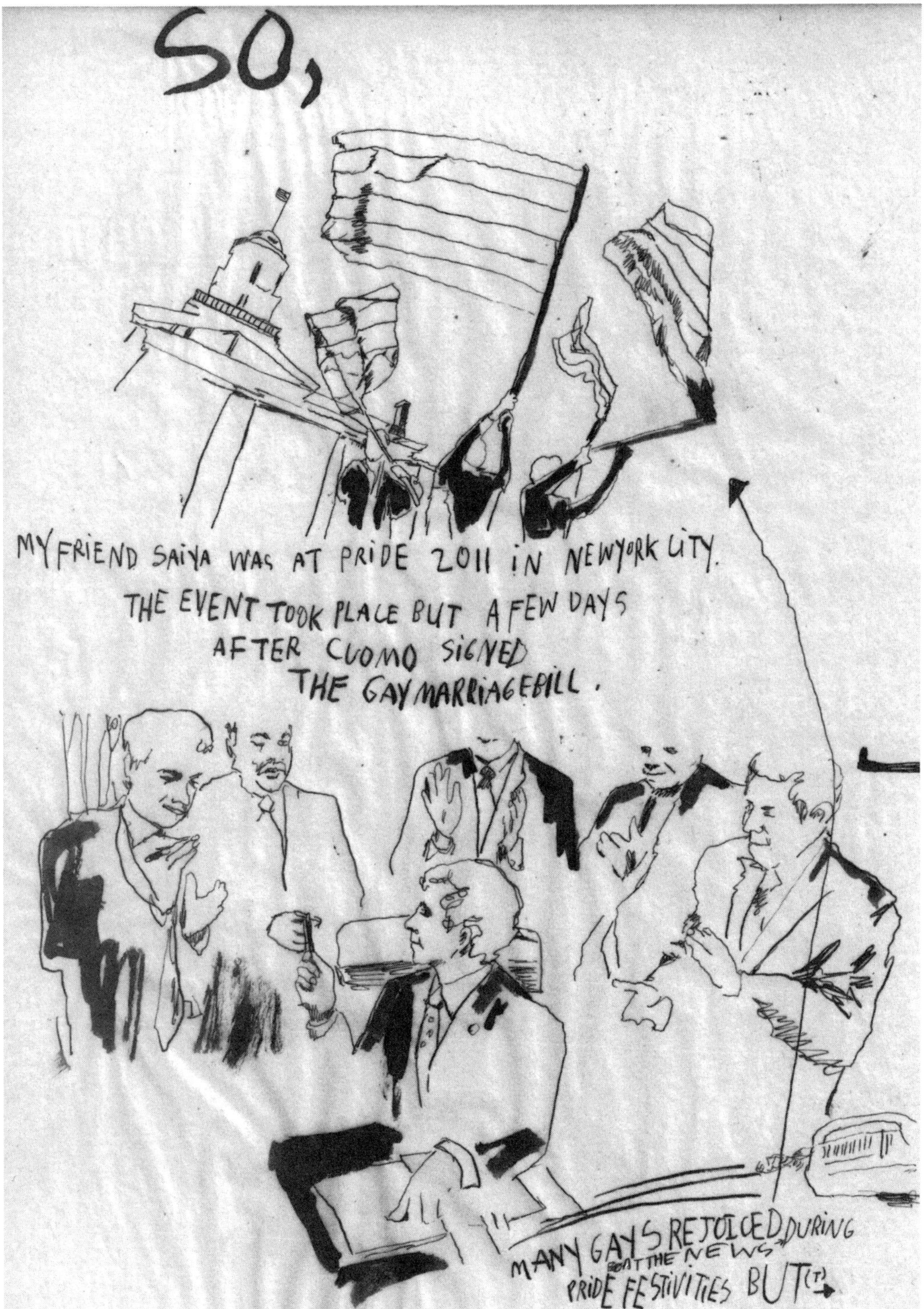
SO,
MY FRIEND SAIYA WAS AT PRIDE 2011 IN NEW YORK CITY.
THE EVENT TOOK PLACE BUT A FEW DAYS
AFTER CUOMO SIGNED
THE GAY MARRIAGE BILL.
MANY GAYS REJOICED DURING
AT THE NEWS
PRIDE FESTIVITIES BUT(T)

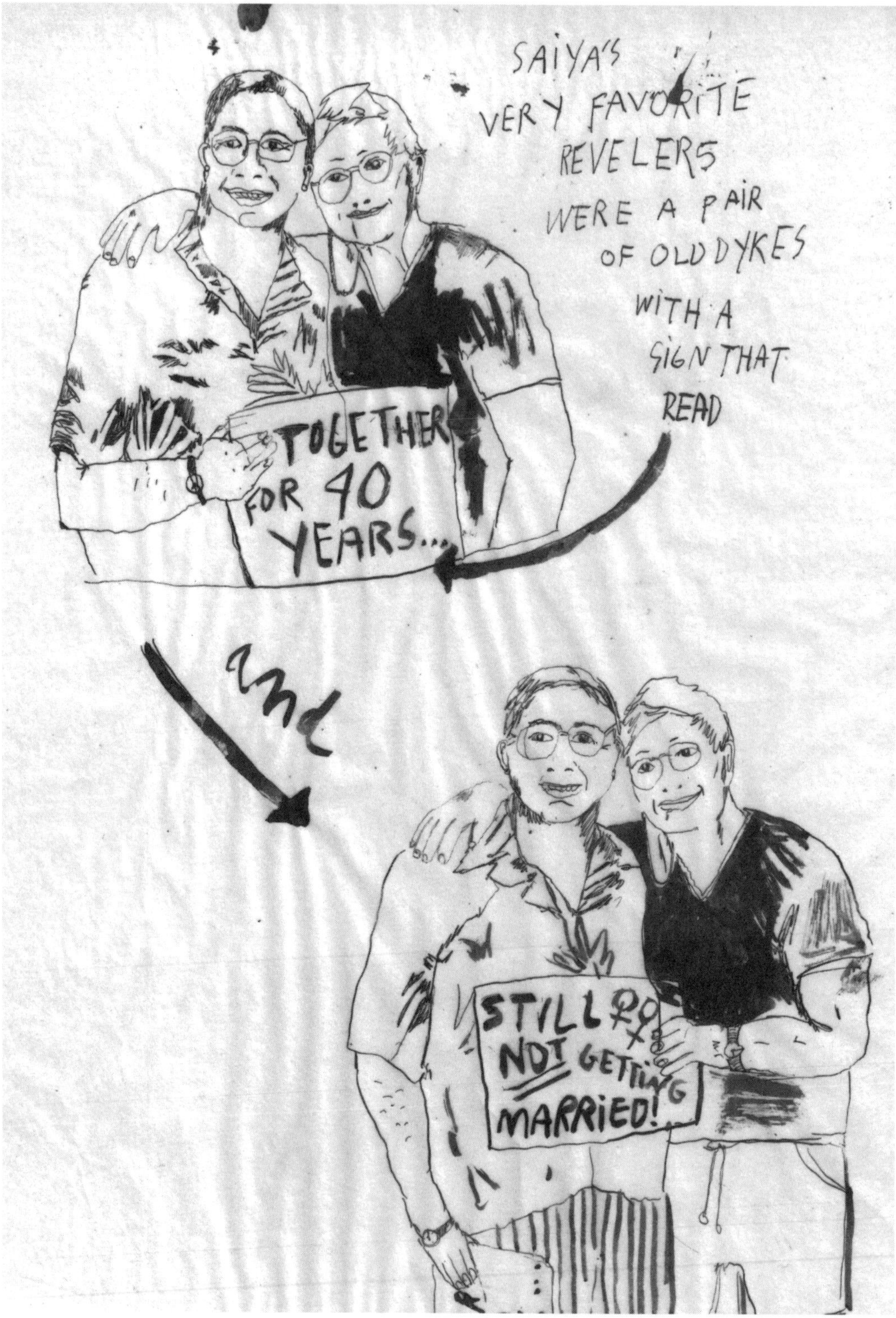
SAIYA'S VERY FAVORITE REVELERS WERE A PAIR OF OLD DYKES WITH A SIGN THAT READ
TOGETHER FOR 40 YEARS...
and
STILL ♀♀ NOT GETTING MARRIED!

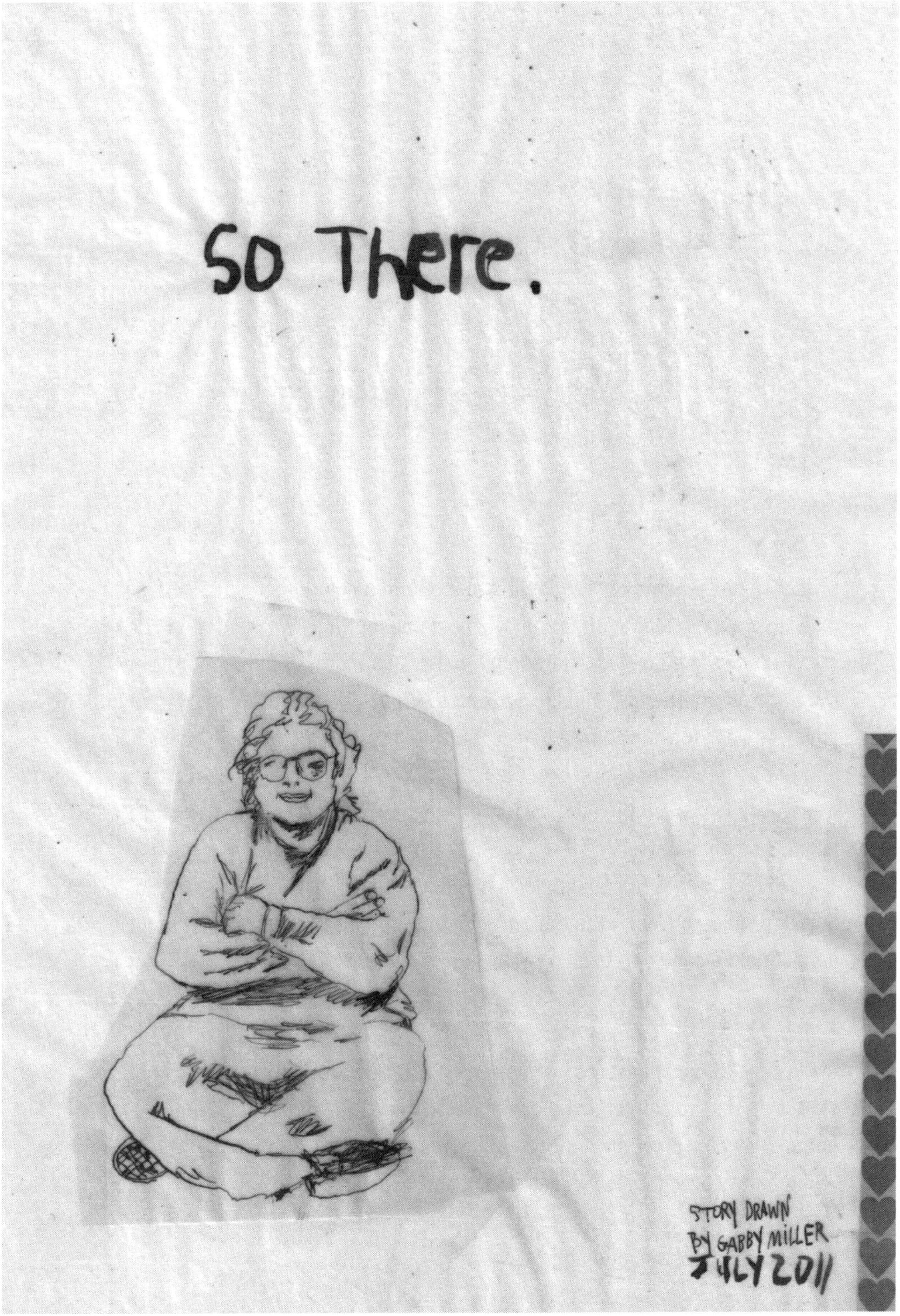
So There.
STORY DRAWN
BY GABBY MILLER
JULY 2011

CHAPTER SIX:

ENDINGS

SAIYA

My sister has a name for the feeling of a doomed relationship. It's called breakup belly. It is a deep feeling that something is nauseatingly wrong. It sits heavy and cold in your stomach, like fried dough eaten in a moment of blind excitement at the fair. You ate the funnel cake, which was delicious and hot and greasy, and the sugar powdered your chin and nose, and then you jumped on the roller coaster and put up your arms and screamed, "WOOOO!" The lights were dazzling and everything was spinning, and then the ride slowly came to a halt and you just did not feel so good anymore.

When it comes to making decisions in relationships, sometimes the belly is a better indicator than even the purest logic. All the sound reasoning in the world cannot hold a candle to trusting your gut.

LIZA

My first relationship started when I was fourteen. Alex was a curly-haired skateboarder and I fell hard. Our connectedness was extreme. My identity was completely consumed by Alex. One plus one equaled one. I held my breath and my tongue, worried that I would exhale and he would be gone. Unfortunately, this worry was unfounded: Alex never left. Even though he ended the relationship over a decade ago, his residue lingers.

He took advantage of my desire to be loved. There were many conditions I had to meet to earn his love. One was being able to accept that my jealousy drove Alex to flirt with our classmates and my friends. I also had to believe his lies. He lied about everything, just to hear the words. Just as I accepted my grade school friends' teasing, I accepted Alex's abuse, for those infrequent moments of acknowledgment.

He awakened my sexual appetite, but my sexuality was only a tool to unlock his. The only question Alex asked me was, "Does this hurt too much?" He never asked, "Does this feel good?" I wasted a year of my life trying to please him. I never felt safe.

After Alex broke up with me, I spent most of my time wasted in mosh pits, surrounded by the best friends I'll ever have. Beer and liquor were everywhere. Even with my support network, I often found myself drunk and crying at the end of the night, replaying memories from my relationship with Alex. My new partner at the time, Casey, cared for me, cleaned up after me, and listened to my broken-hearted teenage poetry. Despite Casey's innocent love, I was consumed by memories of Alex and my broken trust.

SAIYA

It is obvious that it is hard to say good-bye to a good thing. But it can be surprising when saying good-bye to a bad thing is hard, too. Strange, that the things that hurt the most are the toughest to let go. They give us easy comfort, but not long-term love. They are interesting. They are compelling. They afford a look into the fabric of darkness, which is worth understanding. But ultimately, they have nothing to give back.

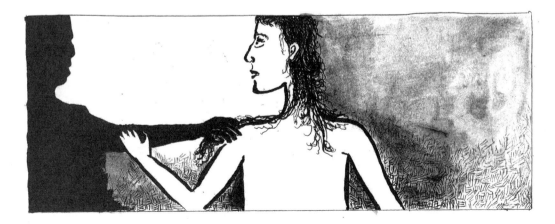

LIZA

With the hindsight of ten years of failed romance, I can see how much of my sexual identity was framed by that pivotal relationship with Alex. Between the sheets I'll perform what I think is expected of me, often sacrificing my own desires, fearing that a misstep or an ill-planned caress will end the entire interaction.

Returning to the narratives in *Not Your Mother's Meatloaf* strengthens my character. Reading others' stories emboldens my sexuality. Communicating my needs during the stumbles and rumbles of passion turns me on, when I'm brave enough to speak up. Reading about our shared histories in our communities is a powerful motivator. The comics remind me that I'm not alone in insecurity, sexual desire, and confusion.

ALEX & ME
JUST ME
I WAS LEFT EMPTY
BUT, MY FRIENDS PICKED ME UP AND NEVER LET GO

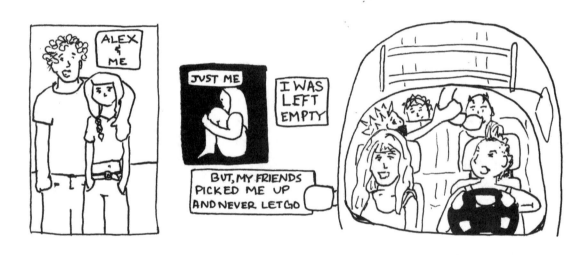

SAIYA

I am picturing a visit that I might pay to my younger self. Like a genie, I would take my hand and begin to explain. For every bad habit, for each lousy person that you let go of, you will receive something precious and new. Instead of that sneaky friend who lies to and uses you, you will find a group of the most loving, interesting, and inspiring people. Here, instead of eating little besides potato chips for lunch in the girls' room, you will feast on whatever you like in good company. Instead of this guy, who is leeching out all of your energy and still begging for more, you can have your independence and your freedom. You will have other lovers. Each one will teach you something new. Stop playing with that bloody baby tooth. Just tie it to a doorknob, yank it out, and make room. When you wake up, there will be something better under your pillow. When the new tooth comes in, it is going to be stronger and better at chewing anyway.

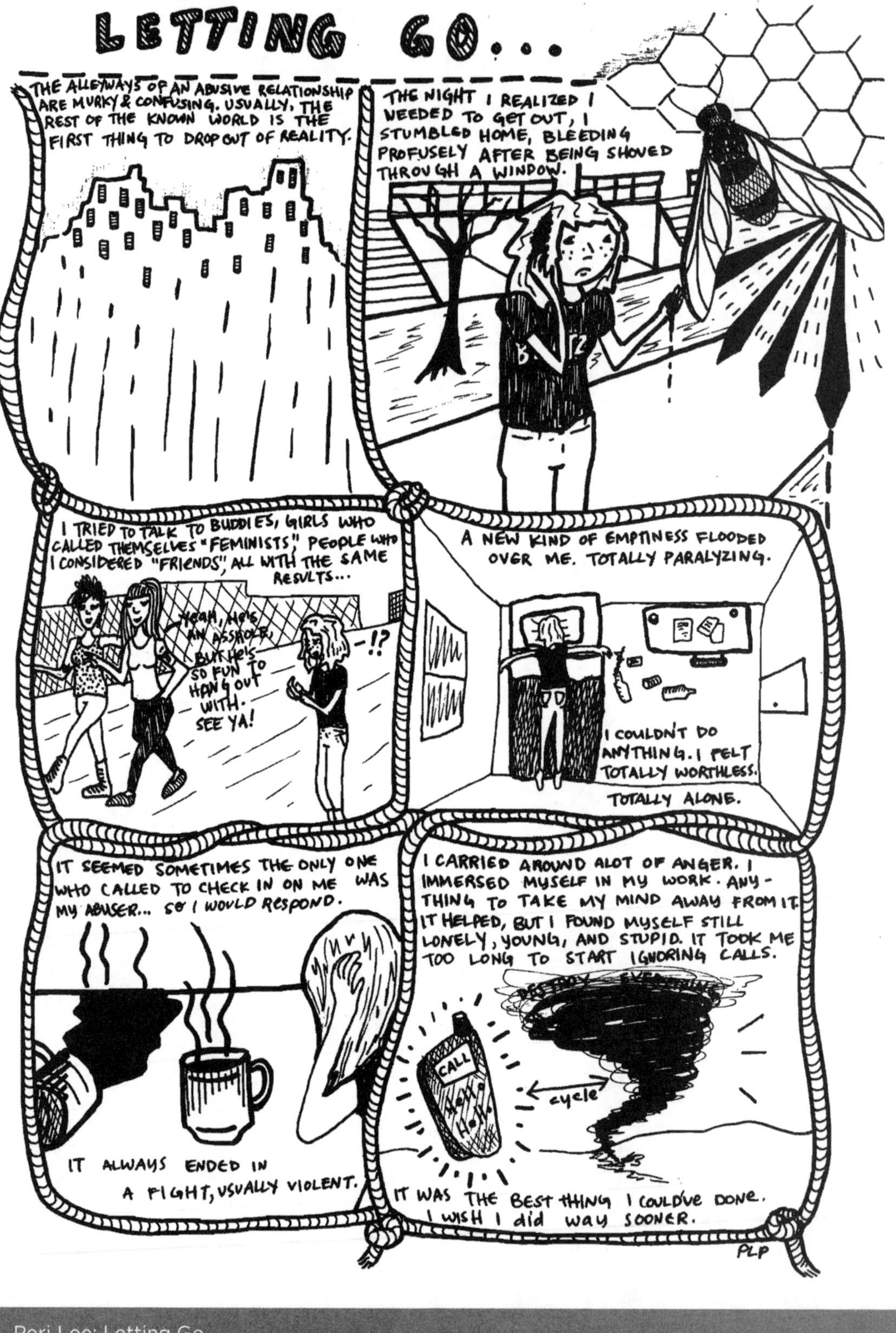
LETTING GO...
THE ALLEYWAYS OF AN ABUSIVE RELATIONSHIP ARE MURKY & CONFUSING. USUALLY, THE REST OF THE KNOWN WORLD IS THE FIRST THING TO DROP OUT OF REALITY.
THE NIGHT I REALIZED I NEEDED TO GET OUT, I STUMBLED HOME, BLEEDING PROFUSELY AFTER BEING SHOVED THROUGH A WINDOW.
I TRIED TO TALK TO BUDDIES, GIRLS WHO CALLED THEMSELVES "FEMINISTS," PEOPLE WHO I CONSIDERED "FRIENDS," ALL WITH THE SAME RESULTS...
YEAH, HE'S AN ASSHOLE, BUT HE'S SO FUN TO HANG OUT WITH. SEE YA!
-!?
A NEW KIND OF EMPTINESS FLOODED OVER ME. TOTALLY PARALYZING.
I COULDN'T DO ANYTHING. I FELT TOTALLY WORTHLESS.
TOTALLY ALONE.
IT SEEMED SOMETIMES THE ONLY ONE WHO CALLED TO CHECK IN ON ME WAS MY ABUSER... SO I WOULD RESPOND.
IT ALWAYS ENDED IN A FIGHT, USUALLY VIOLENT.
I CARRIED AROUND ALOT OF ANGER. I IMMERSED MYSELF IN MY WORK. ANYTHING TO TAKE MY MIND AWAY FROM IT. IT HELPED, BUT I FOUND MYSELF STILL LONELY, YOUNG, AND STUPID. IT TOOK ME TOO LONG TO START IGNORING CALLS.
CALL
cycle
IT WAS THE BEST THING I COULD'VE DONE. I WISH I did way SOONER.
PLP

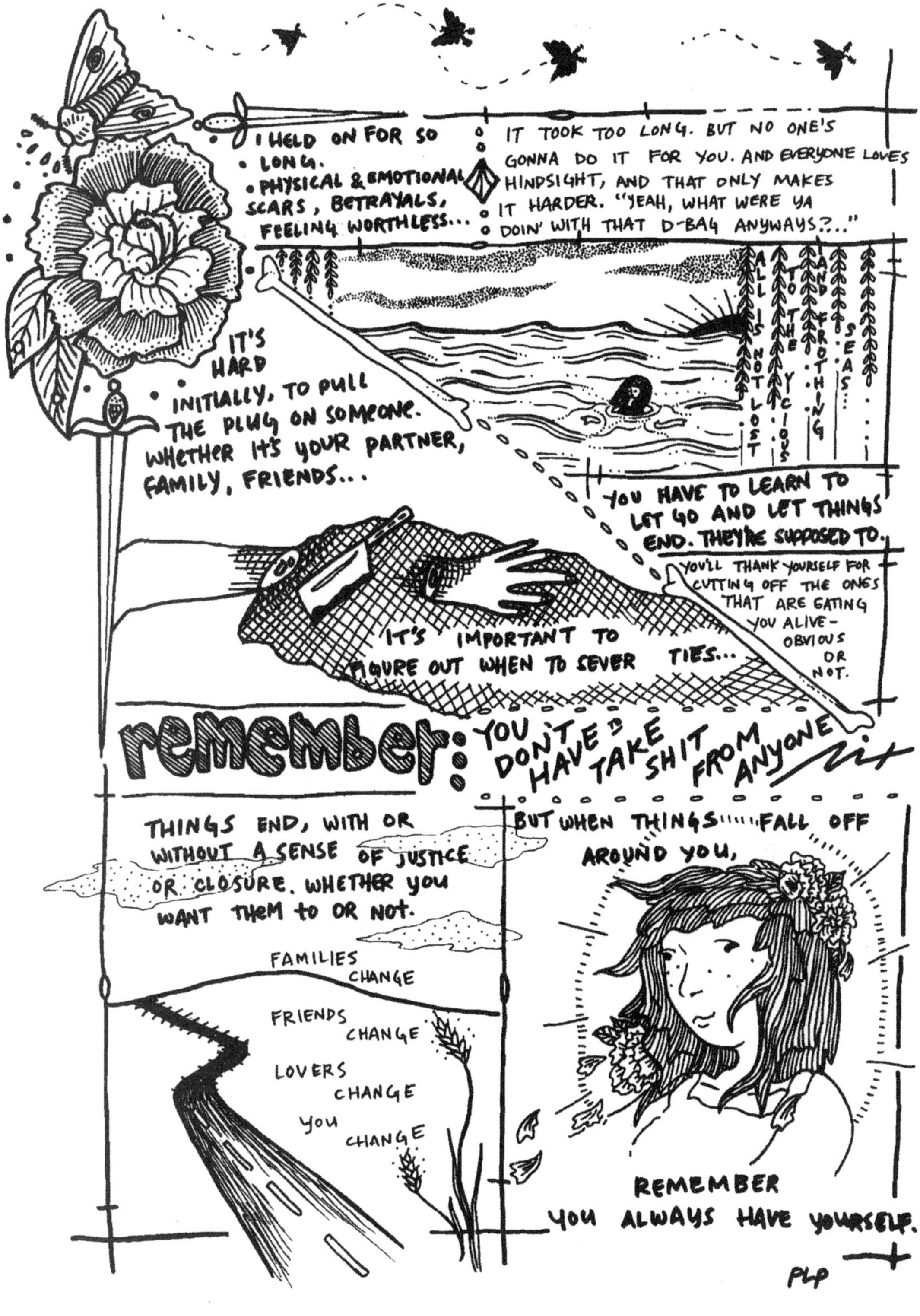
I HELD ON FOR SO LONG.
PHYSICAL & EMOTIONAL SCARS, BETRAYALS, FEELING WORTHLESS...
IT TOOK TOO LONG. BUT NO ONE'S GONNA DO IT FOR YOU. AND EVERYONE LOVES HINDSIGHT, AND THAT ONLY MAKES IT HARDER. "YEAH, WHAT WERE YA DOIN' WITH THAT D-BAG ANYWAYS?..."
ALL IS NOT LOST
TO THE VICIOUS
AND FROTHING
SEAS...
IT'S HARD INITIALLY, TO PULL THE PLUG ON SOMEONE. WHETHER IT'S YOUR PARTNER, FAMILY, FRIENDS...
YOU HAVE TO LEARN TO LET GO AND LET THINGS END. THEY'RE SUPPOSED TO.
YOU'LL THANK YOURSELF FOR CUTTING OFF THE ONES THAT ARE EATING YOU ALIVE - OBVIOUS OR NOT.
IT'S IMPORTANT TO FIGURE OUT WHEN TO SEVER TIES...
remember: YOU DON'T HAVE TO TAKE SHIT FROM ANYONE
THINGS END, WITH OR WITHOUT A SENSE OF JUSTICE OR CLOSURE. WHETHER YOU WANT THEM TO OR NOT.
FAMILIES CHANGE
FRIENDS CHANGE
LOVERS CHANGE
YOU CHANGE
BUT WHEN THINGS FALL OFF AROUND YOU,
REMEMBER YOU ALWAYS HAVE YOURSELF.
PLP

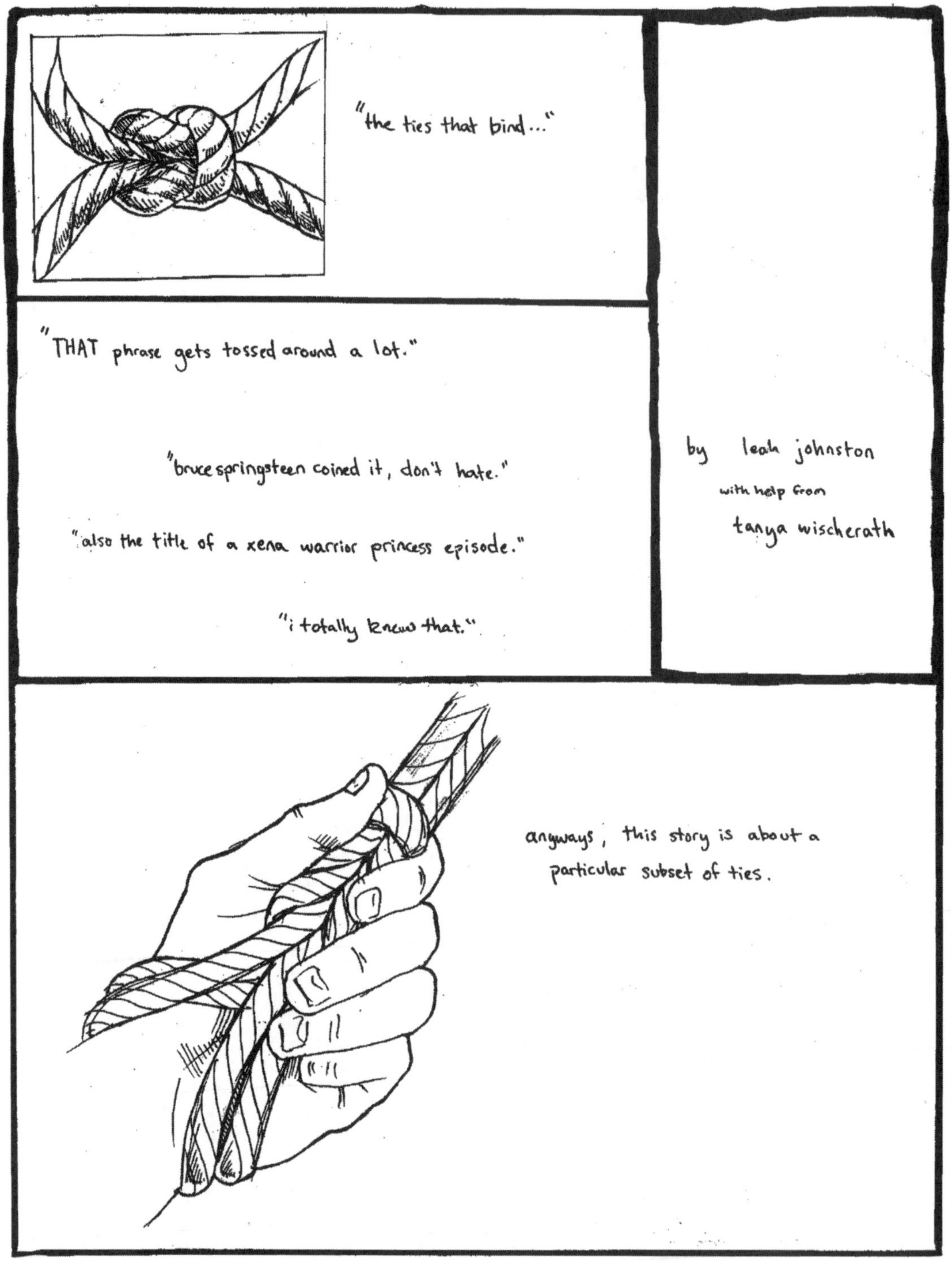
"the ties that bind..."
"THAT phrase gets tossed around a lot."
"bruce springsteen coined it, don't hate."
"also the title of a xena warrior princess episode."
"i totally know that."
by leah johnston
with help from
tanya wischerath
anyways, this story is about a particular subset of ties.

ah.

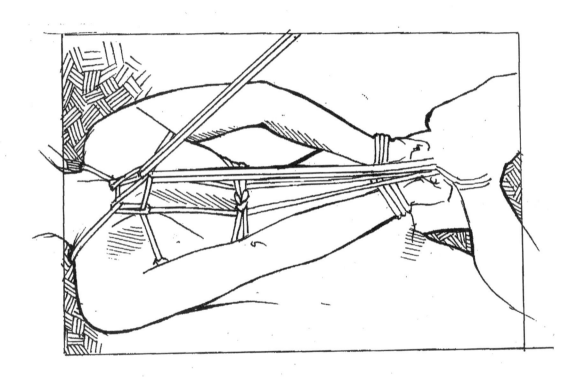

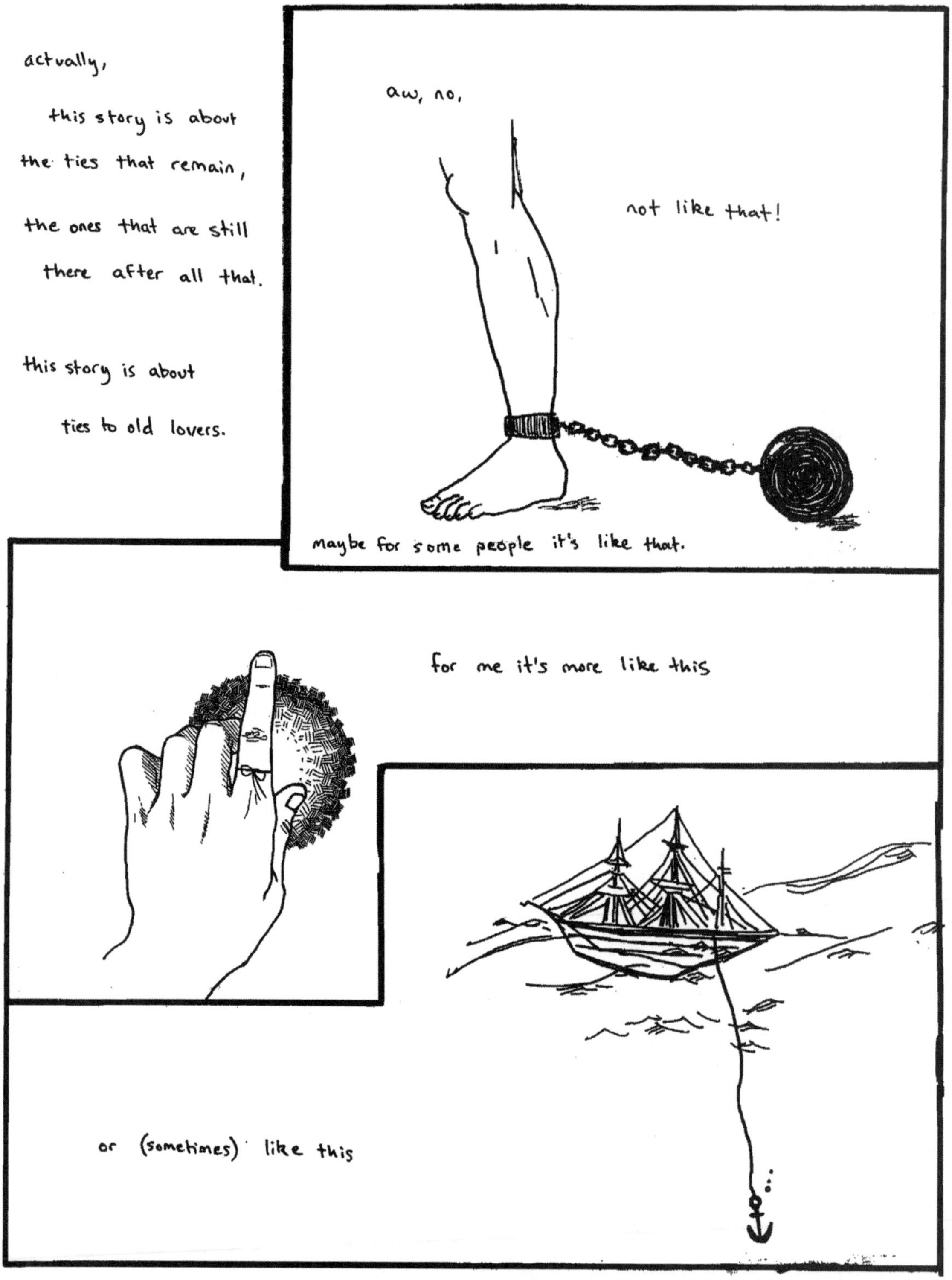

actually,

this story is about the ties that remain, the ones that are still there after all that.

this story is about ties to old lovers.

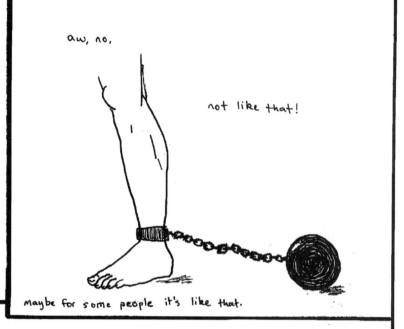

aw, no,

not like that!

maybe for some people it's like that.

for me it's more like this

or (sometimes) like this

people can be connected in a myriad of ways i guess, but in my experience physical intimacy creates a very clear set of bonds.

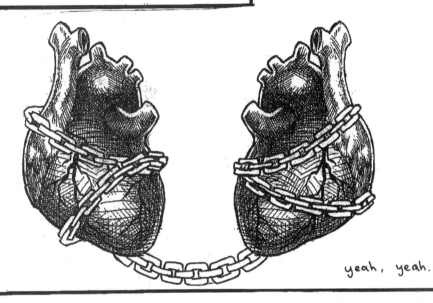

yeah, yeah.

they're not all the same, they're characteristic to you and your lover, just like your gorgeous snowflake self.

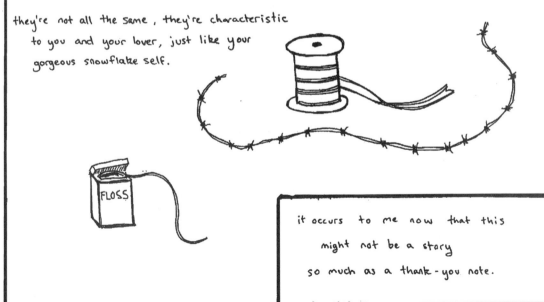

FLOSS

it occurs to me now that this might not be a story so much as a thank-you note.

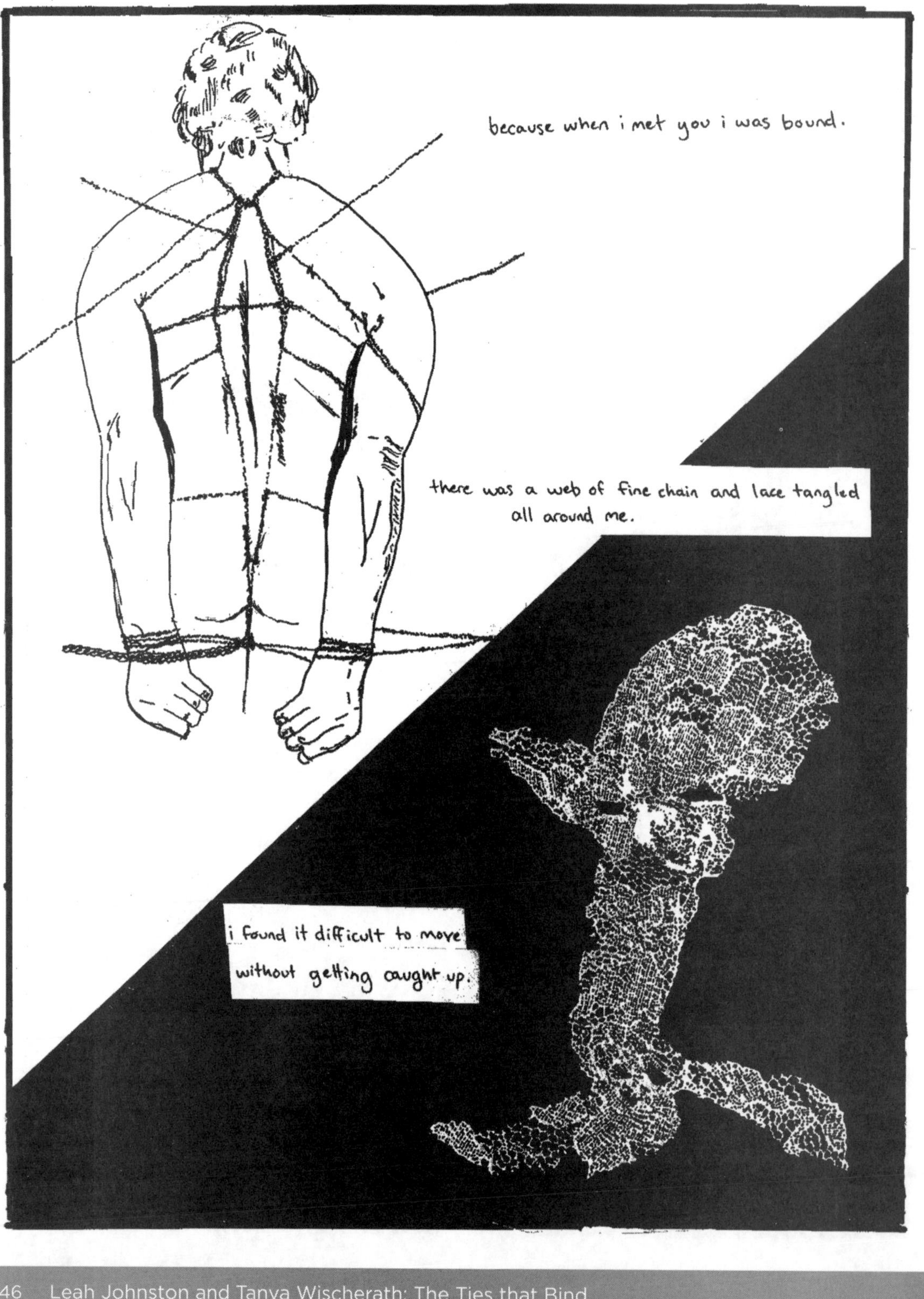
because when i met you i was bound.
there was a web of fine chain and lace tangled all around me.
i found it difficult to move
without getting caught up.

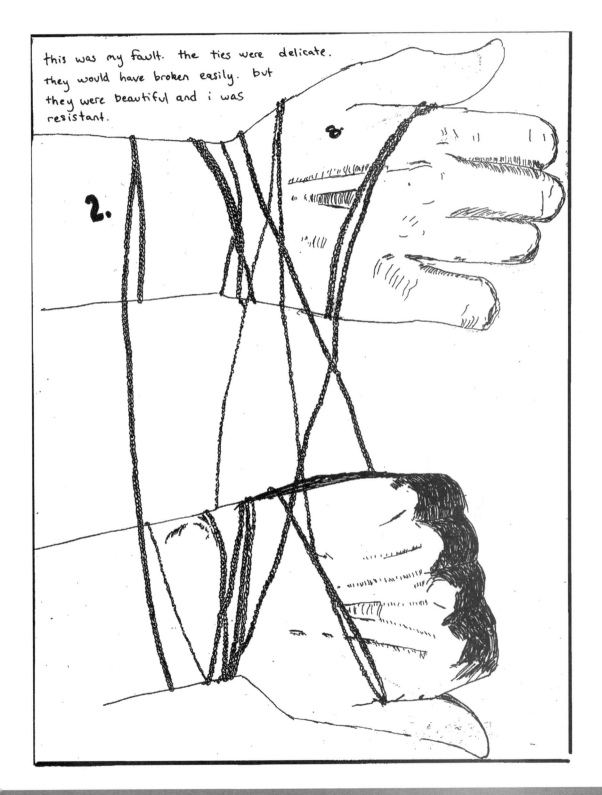

this was my fault. the ties were delicate.
they would have broken easily. but
they were beautiful and i was
resistant.

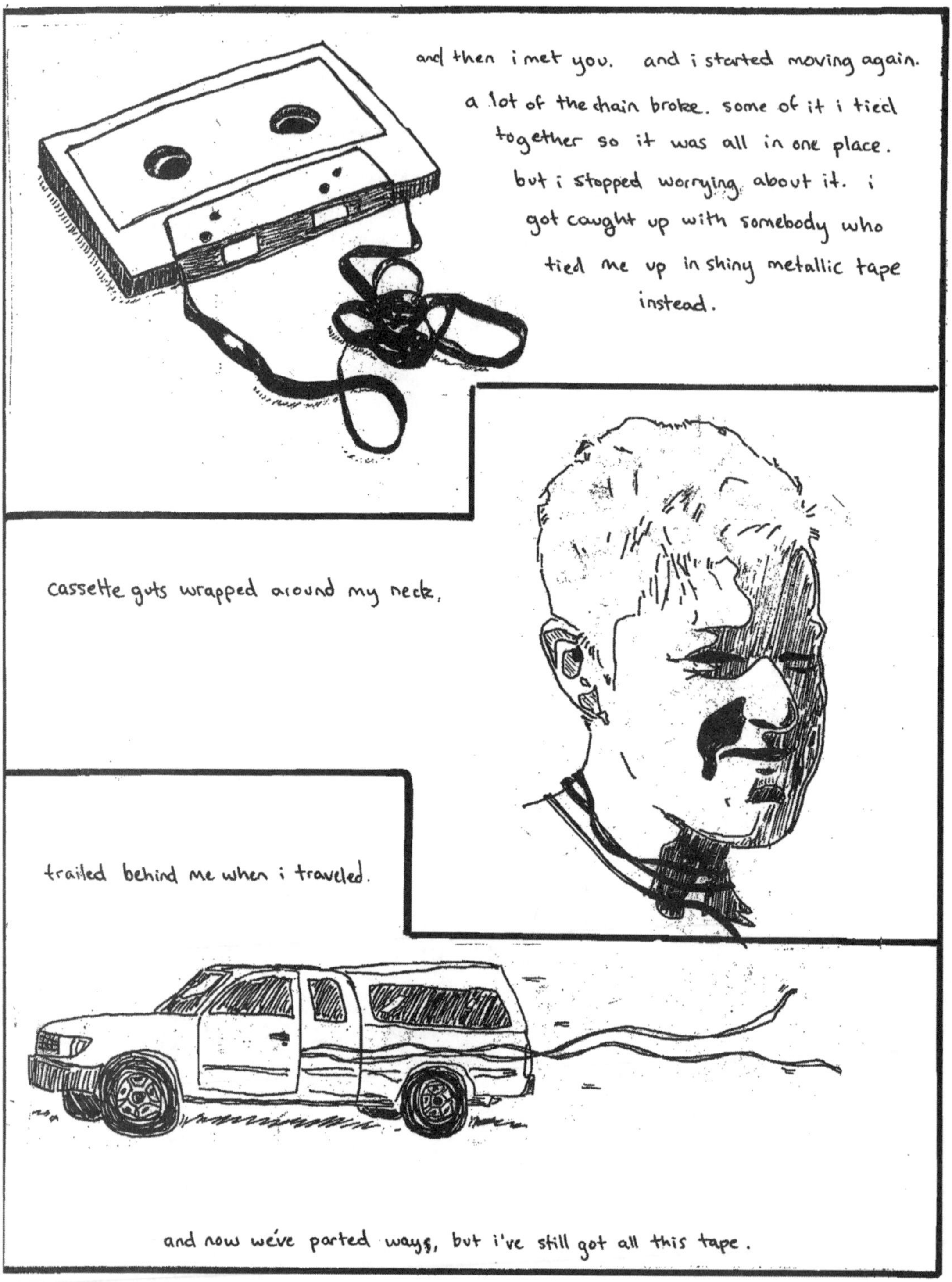
and then i met you. and i started moving again.
a lot of the chain broke. some of it i tied together so it was all in one place. but i stopped worrying about it. i got caught up with somebody who tied me up in shiny metallic tape instead.
cassette guts wrapped around my neck,
trailed behind me when i traveled.
and now we've parted ways, but i've still got all this tape.

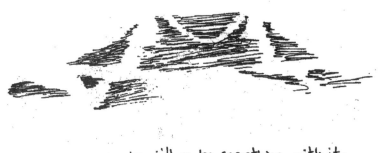

maybe i'll make something with it.

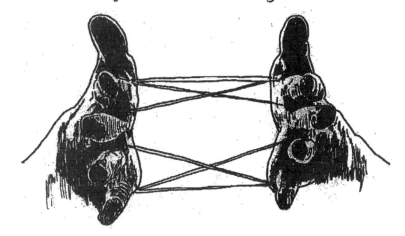

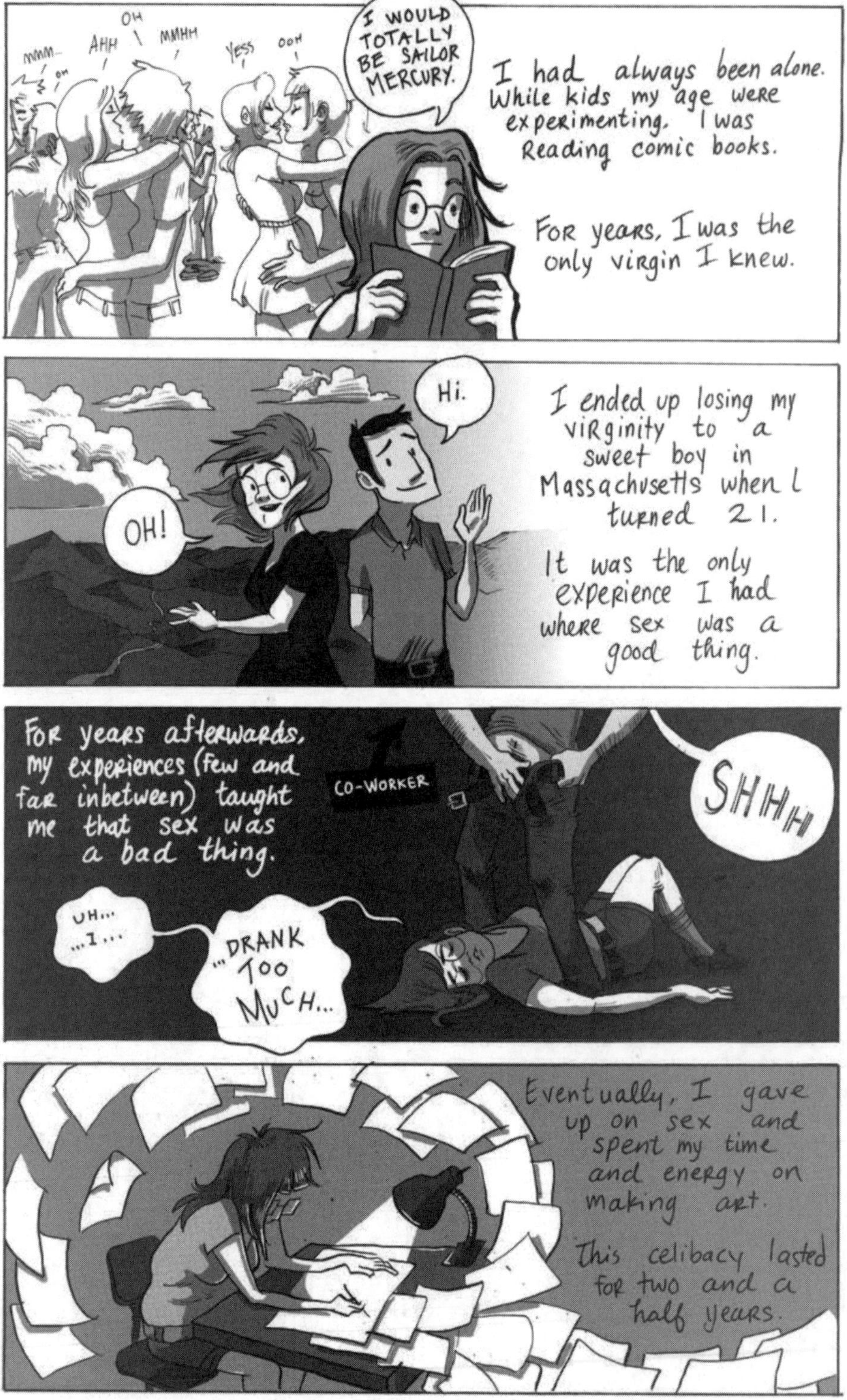
mmm
oh
AHH
OH
MMHH
Yess
OOH
I WOULD TOTALLY BE SAILOR MERCURY.
I had always been alone. While kids my age were experimenting, I was Reading comic books.
For years, I was the only virgin I knew.
Hi.
OH!
I ended up losing my virginity to a sweet boy in Massachusetts when I turned 21.
It was the only experience I had where sex was a good thing.
For years afterwards, my experiences (few and far inbetween) taught me that sex was a bad thing.
CO-WORKER
SHHH
UH… …I…
…DRANK TOO MUCH…
Eventually, I gave up on sex and spent my time and energy on making art.
This celibacy lasted for two and a half years.

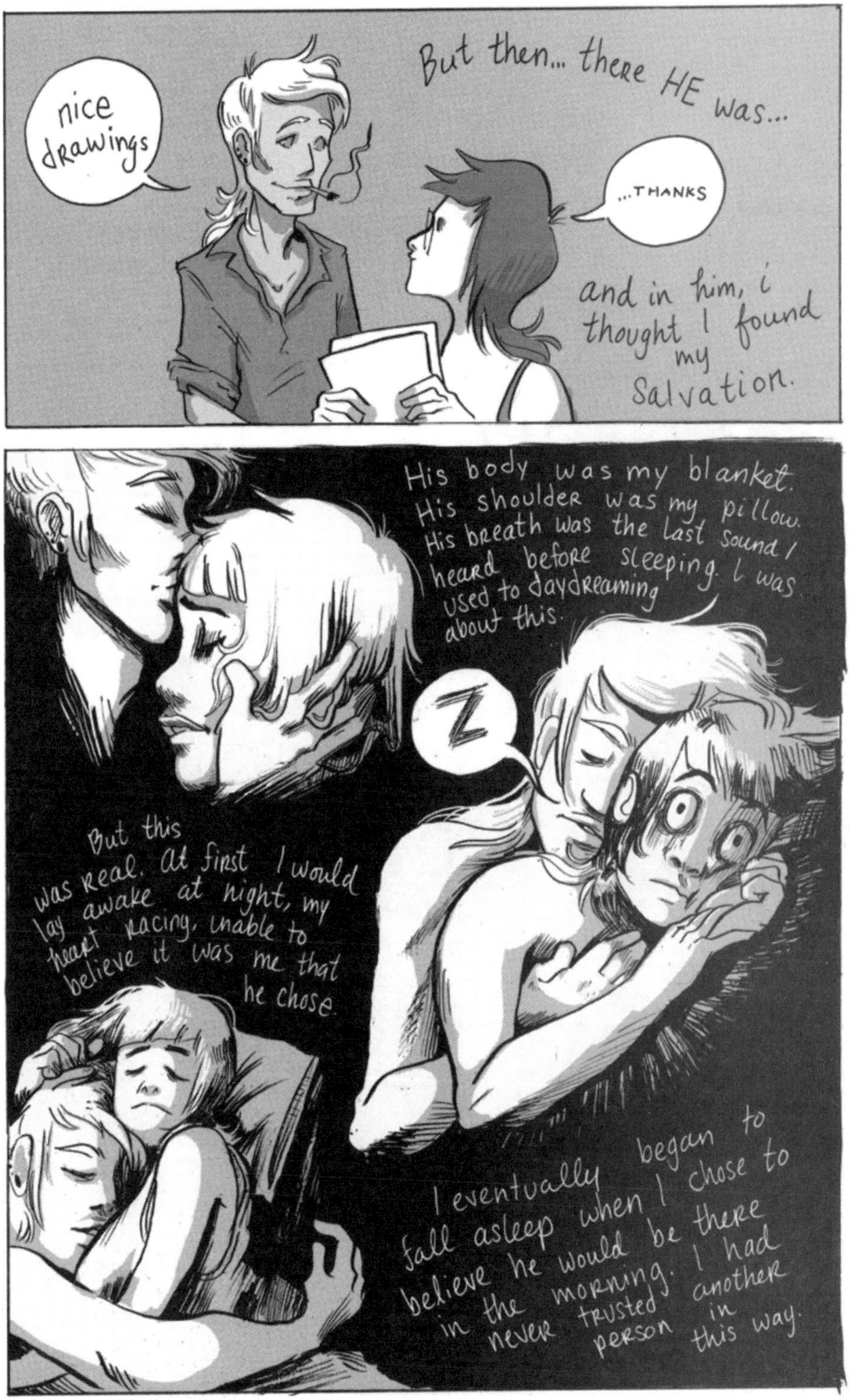
But then... there HE was...
nice drawings
...THANKS
and in him, i thought I found my Salvation.
His body was my blanket. His shoulder was my pillow. His breath was the last sound I heard before sleeping. I was used to daydreaming about this.
Z
But this was real. At first I would lay awake at night, my heart racing, unable to believe it was me that he chose.
I eventually began to fall asleep when I chose to believe he would be there in the morning. I had never trusted another person in this way.

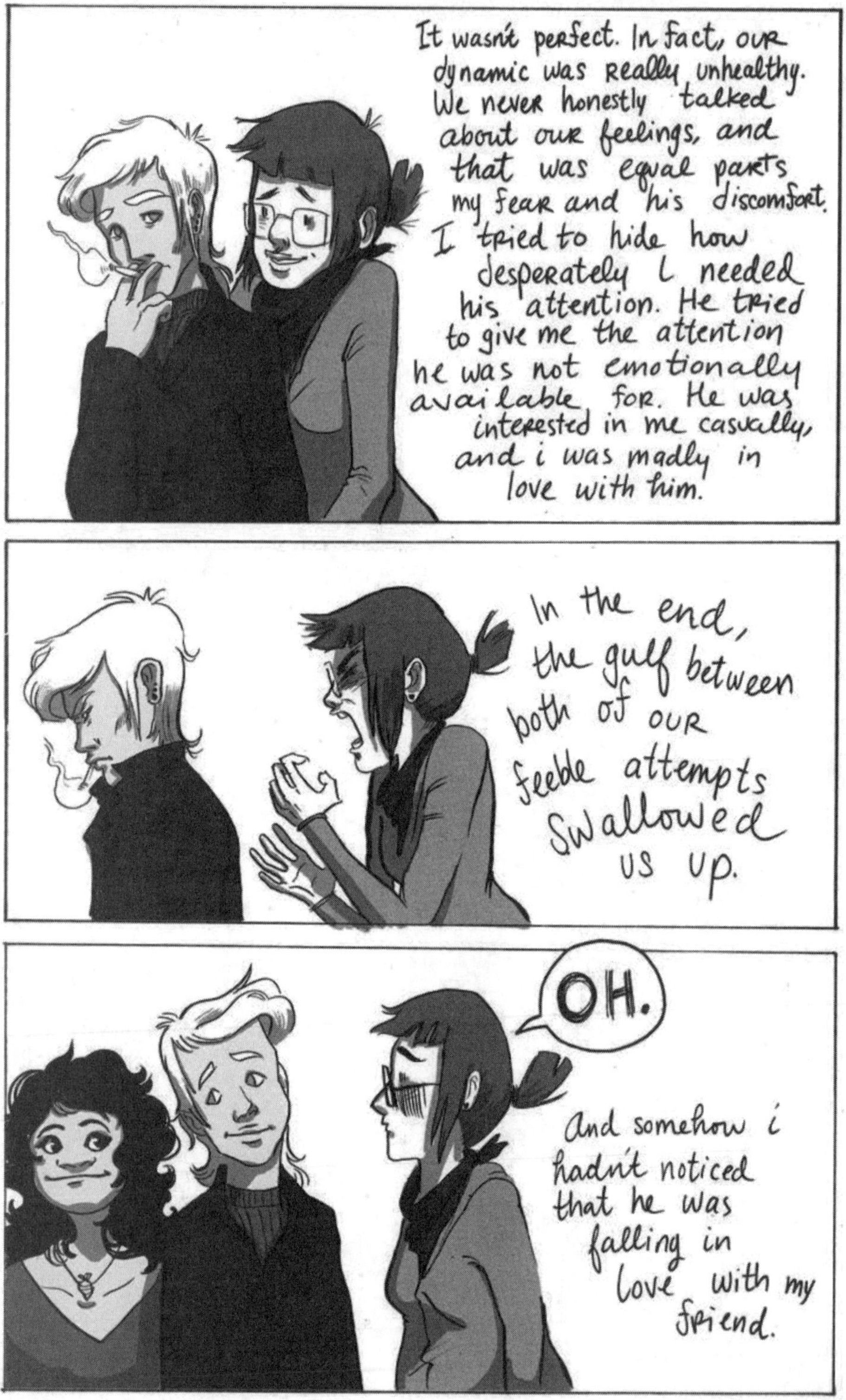
It wasn't perfect. In fact, our dynamic was really unhealthy. We never honestly talked about our feelings, and that was equal parts my fear and his discomfort. I tried to hide how desperately I needed his attention. He tried to give me the attention he was not emotionally available for. He was interested in me casually, and i was madly in love with him.
In the end, the gulf between both of our feeble attempts swallowed us up.
OH.
And somehow i hadn't noticed that he was falling in love with my friend.

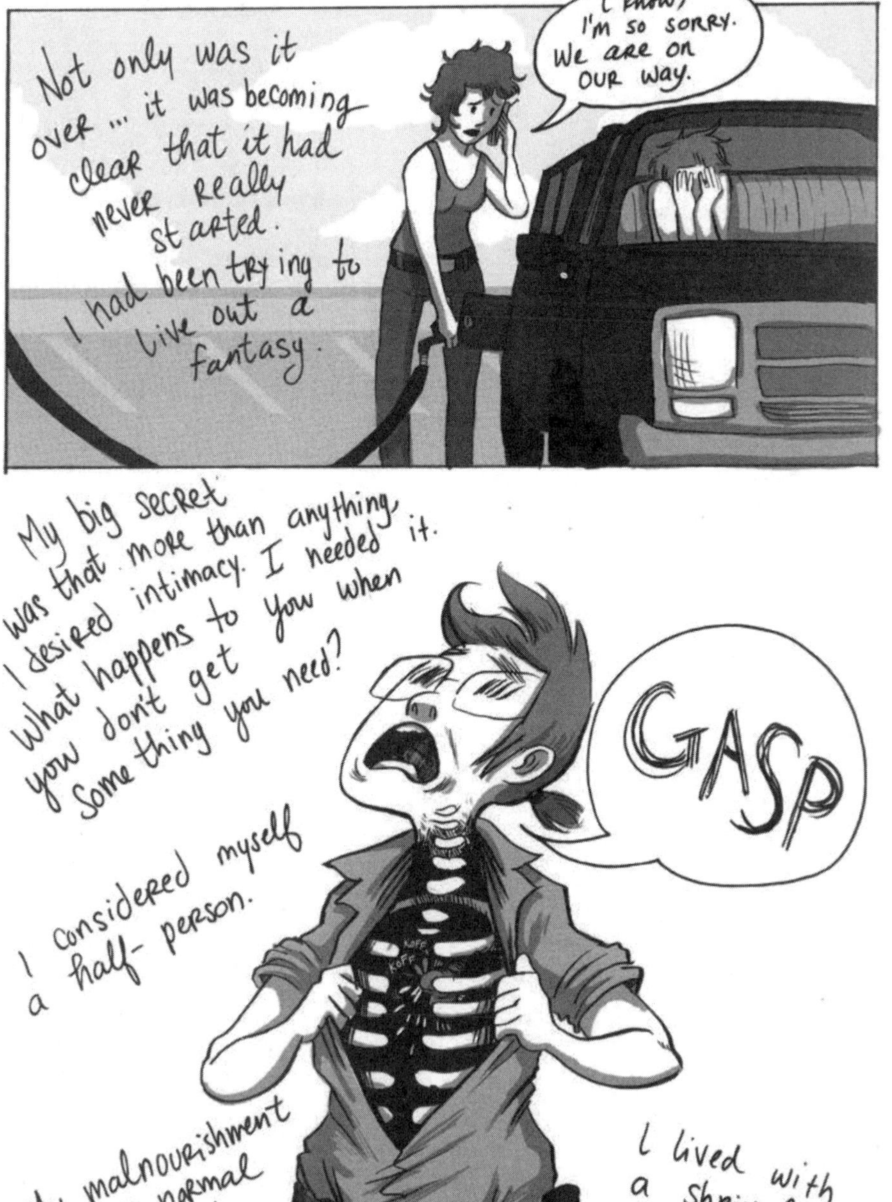
Not only was it over ... it was becoming clear that it had never really started.
I had been trying to live out a fantasy.
I know, I'm so sorry. We are on our way.
My big secret was that more than anything, I desired intimacy. I needed it.
What happens to you when you don't get something you need?
GASP
I considered myself a half-person.
My malnourishment was so normal to me that I had never noticed...
I lived with a shriveled up heart.

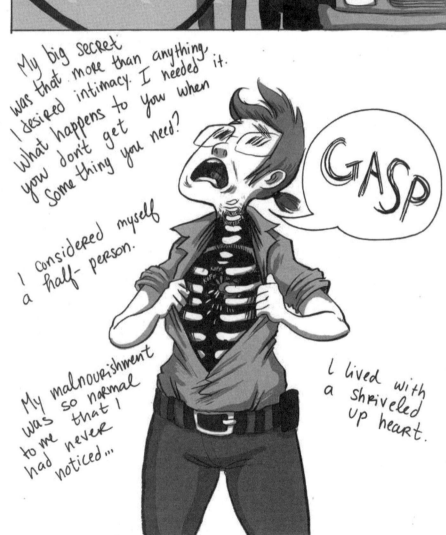

I awoke with a tingling sensation on my lip. Felt kinda like when you get peppermint Bronners on yer butthole... ya know?

And then I looked in the mirror...
"WHAT THE FUCK! IS THAT HERPES?"
... there was a cluster of little red bumbs below my lower lip.

So this is it...

The End

...of my sex life.

I went to the local coffee shop to research oral herpes. I had my hat pulled low & my hood up. I wasn't even in a town where I knew anyone, but the social stigma was all ready hitting me hard.

The first image search confirmed it. I freaked out. I cursed the last random person I made out with. I cursed myself for being promiscuous. I mourned the lovers I was bound to lose and I mentally started to prepare myself for a monk-like life of solitude & chastity. And then I continued my research.

Some Things I Learned.*

- Most HSV-1 (#2 is genital herpes) infections happen in the hospital as we're infants. (So I could have had this my whole life and shouldn't blame anyone, including myself.)
- "Outbreaks" can be triggered by stress, ultraviolet light (sunshine), heat, fatigue, immune depression, etc. (I'd been extremely stressed, working hard out in the hot sun for prolonged periods. This was making sense.)
- Sometime between the ages of 14 & 49 60% of the population will be infected with HSV-1. By 80 its like 90%. However, only about 30% will ever show signs of infection.
- Oral herpes is highly contagious during outbreaks, and scientist believe it is possible to spread even when there is no sign of outbreak. (Hence, everyone & their mother having it.)

* this is all stuff I pulled off the web. please do your own research if you think you have any S.T.I.

An infant.

The Sun.

me workin' hard.

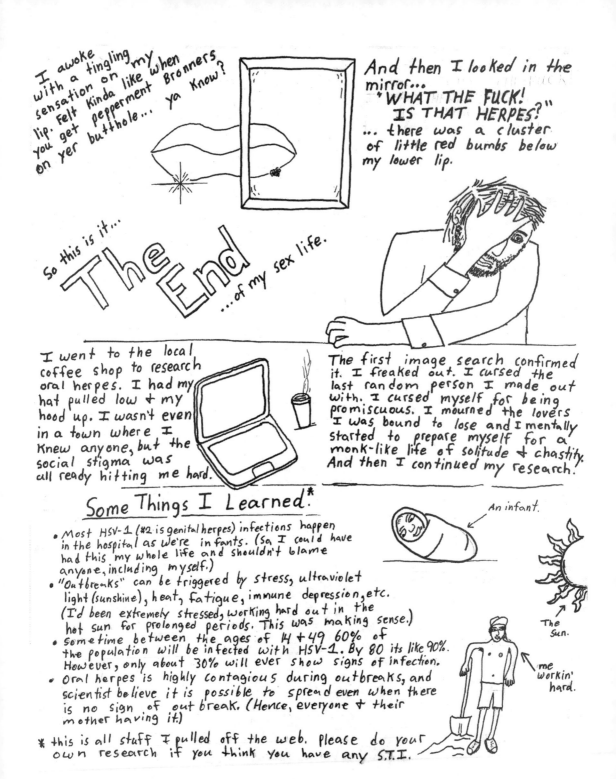

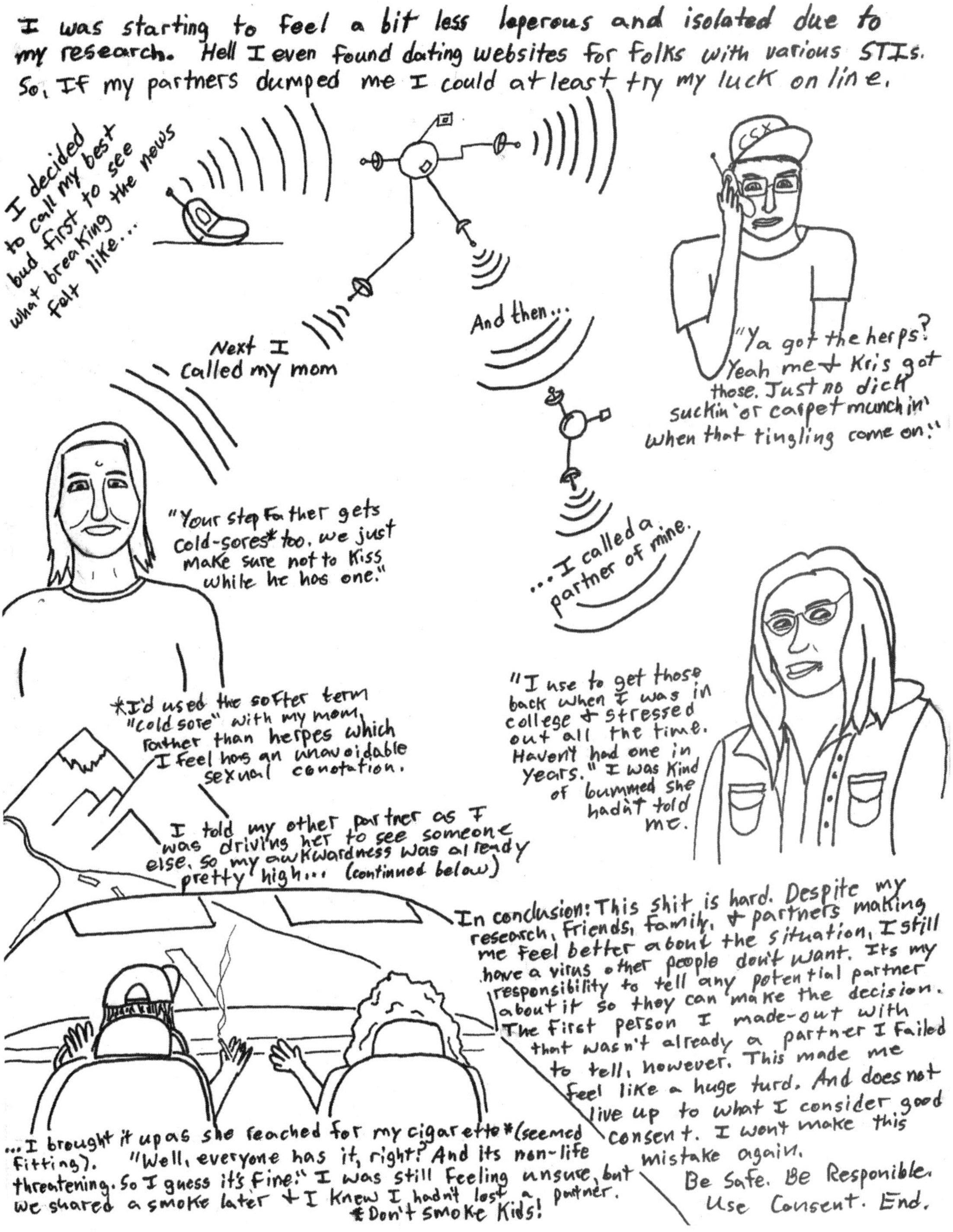
I was starting to feel a bit less leperous and isolated due to my research. Hell I even found dating websites for folks with various STIs. So, If my partners dumped me I could at least try my luck on line.
I decided to call my best bud first to see what breaking the news felt like...
CSX
"Ya got the herps? Yeah me + Kris got those. Just no dick suckin' or carpet munchin' when that tingling come on!"
Next I called my mom
"Your step father gets cold-sores* too. we just make sure not to kiss while he has one."
And then...
...I called a partner of mine.
"I use to get those back when I was in college + stressed out all the time. Haven't had one in years." I was kind of bummed she hadn't told me.
*I'd used the softer term "cold sore" with my mom, rather than herpes which I feel has an unavoidable sexual conotation.
I told my other partner as I was driving her to see someone else, so my awkwardness was already pretty high... (continued below)
...I brought it up as she reached for my cigarette*(seemed fitting). "Well, everyone has it, right? And its non-life threatening. So I guess it's fine." I was still feeling unsure, but we shared a smoke later + I knew I hadn't lost a partner.
*Don't smoke kids!
In conclusion: This shit is hard. Despite my research, friends, family, + partners making me feel better about the situation, I still have a virus other people don't want. Its my responsibility to tell any potential partner about it so they can make the decision. The first person I made-out with that wasn't already a partner I failed to tell, however. This made me feel like a huge turd. And does not live up to what I consider good consent. I won't make this mistake again.
Be Safe. Be Responible. Use Consent. End.

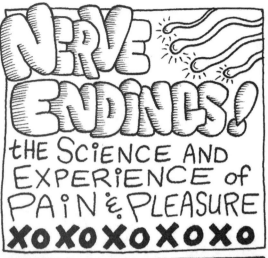

NERVE ENDINGS!
THE SCIENCE AND EXPERIENCE of PAIN & PLEASURE
XO XO XO XO XO XO

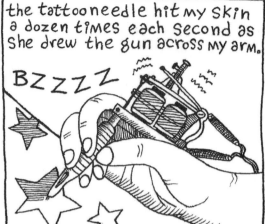

the tattoo needle hit my skin a dozen times each second as she drew the gun across my arm.

BZZZZ

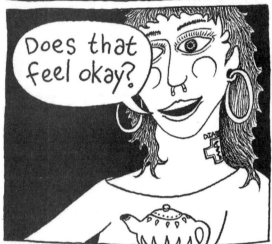

Does that feel okay?

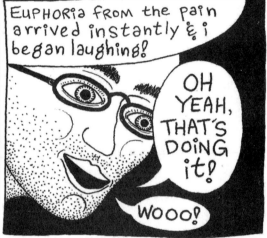

Euphoria from the pain arrived instantly & i began laughing!

OH YEAH, THAT'S DOING it!

WOOO!

After a long while my muscles began twitching & i remembered a time recently when i experienced this twitching after an orgasm. My nerve endings were being stimulated to the maximum, into a state of shock!

How could pain & pleasure be so similar? Science says that orgasm & pain cause the release of similar hormones & chemicals in the body. Science also says that some of these neural pathways in the brain for pain & pleasure are overlapping.

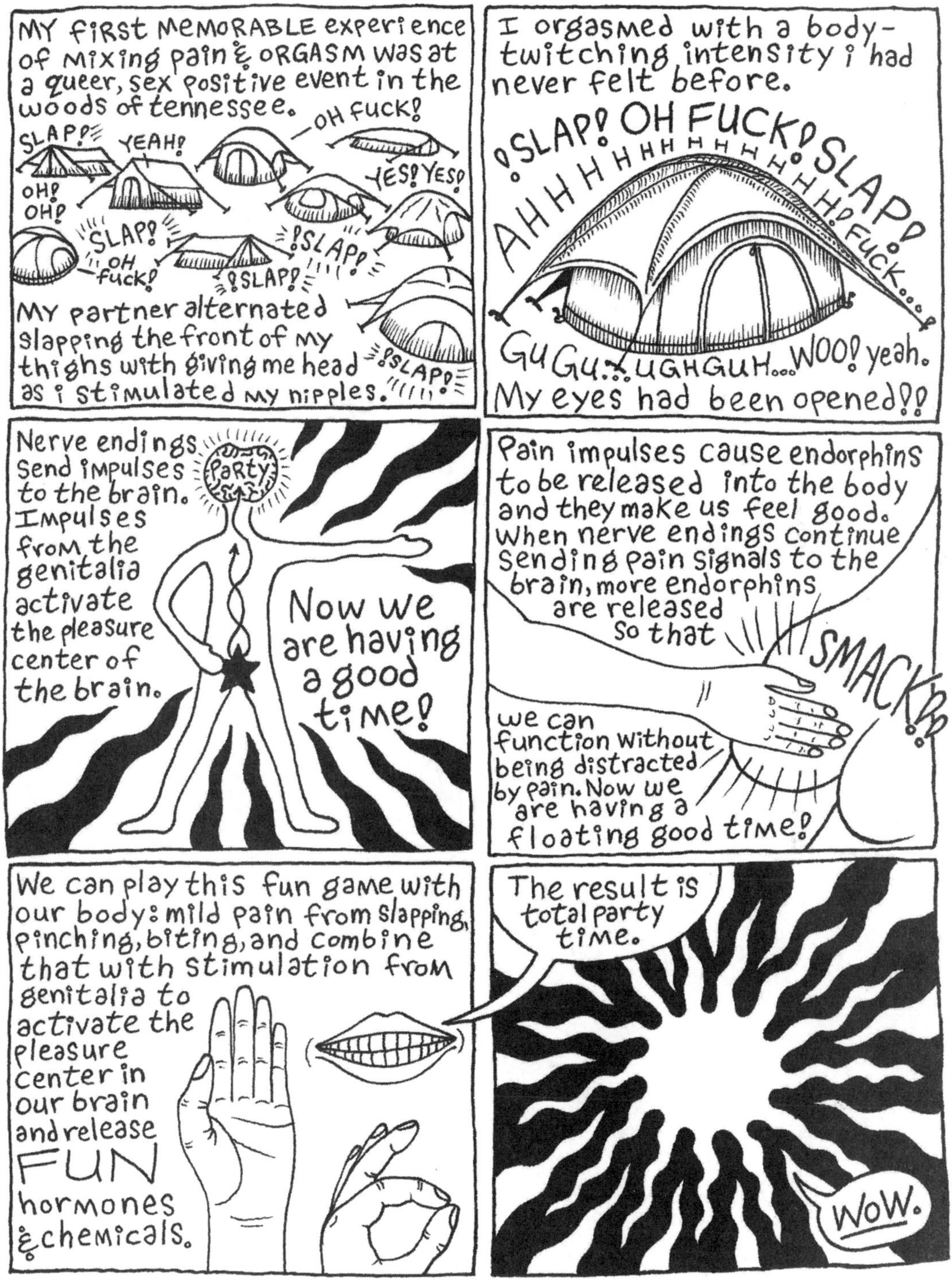
MY first MEMORABLE experience of MIXING pain & ORGASM was at a queer, sex positive event in the woods of tennessee.
SLAP!
YEAH!
OH FUCK!
YES! YES!
OH! OH!
SLAP!
OH fuck!
!SLAP!
!SLAP!
My partner alternated slapping the front of my thighs with giving me head as i stimulated my nipples.
!SLAP!
I orgasmed with a body-twitching intensity i had never felt before.
!SLAP! OH FUCK! SLAP!
AHHHHHHHHHHHHHHH! FUCK...
GUGU...UGHGUH...WOO! yeah.
My eyes had been opened!!
Nerve endings send impulses to the brain. Impulses from the genitalia activate the pleasure center of the brain.
Party
Now we are having a good time!
Pain impulses cause endorphins to be released into the body and they make us feel good. When nerve endings continue sending pain signals to the brain, more endorphins are released so that
SMACK!!
we can function without being distracted by pain. Now we are having a floating good time!
We can play this fun game with our body: mild pain from slapping, pinching, biting, and combine that with stimulation from genitalia to activate the pleasure center in our brain and release FUN hormones & chemicals.
The result is total party time.
WOW.

People who practice BDSM have known this for a long time. It's estimated that about 25% of the U.S. population practices some form of pain & pleasure sexuality.

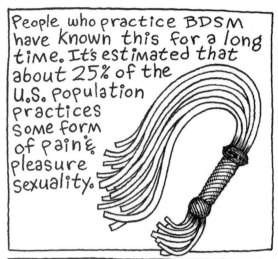

Combining pain techniques with sexual activity has been documented from ancient times in Egypt, INDIA, & Rome.

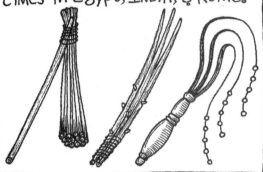

Perhaps ancient people knew many ways to release endorphins and activate the pleasure center:

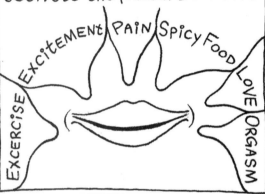

EXERCISE EXCITEMENT PAIN Spicy Food LOVE ORGASM

Different areas of the body have different nerve endings & routes to the brain, resulting in different feelings of pleasure or pain.

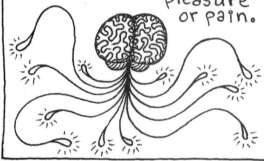

From my experience, i believe we can consciously interpret some signals of pain and choose to feel them as pleasure.

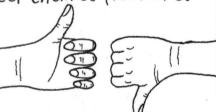

A sexual slap from a lover feels much different than a slap from someone trying to hurt us.

IN OUR amazing bodies we live with incredible potential for pleasure to be unlocked if we, and our lovers, can find the keys.

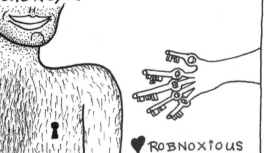

♥ ROBNOXIOUS

CHAPTER SEVEN:

PERSONAL BEST

Our stories did not start with us. Generations have gone before, penciling their confessions, inking in each victory. Bordering on chaos and boxing up the pain, they faced the empty page. In the 1970s, when our parents were just meeting, a San Francisco collective was already putting out *Wimmins Comix*. In 1983, before we were conceived, Rupert Kinnard illustrated queer black narratives. Alison Bechdel warned the public to watch out for dykes when we were in utero. David Wojnarowicz's *7 Miles a Second*, Carl Vaughn Frick's *Watch Out Comix*, and Jaime Cortez's *Sexile* were confronting HIV/AIDS though comics, while the ghosts amassed around them. In the 1990s, as we ran to catch the school bus, the compilation *Dyke Strippers* was released, and Joan Hilty began her tales of a *Bitter Girl*. Ariel Schrag had already drawn her own four-year journey as we awkwardly clawed our way through high school and sprinted out of our hometowns.

YOU HAVE TRICHO-WHAT?
TRICHOMONIASIS
ISN'T THAT FROM RAW PORK?
UM. IT'S AN STI.
1st CALL
HI, HOW ARE, YOU?
WATCH'N REPOMAN
UM, I HAVE TRICH-OMONIASIS
OH, CAN YOU SPELL THAT?
2nd CALL
YEAH I HAVE TRICHOMO-
OH... I HAVE A GIRL FRIEND WANNA HANG OUT?
3rd CALL
I HAVE A STI
I WAS TESTED
OH, OKAY
4th CALL
TRICHOMONIASIS ... YEAH
WE NEVER EXCHANGED FLUIDS
I TOOK ANTIBIOTICS
NO MORE TRICH.
HARD AS IT IS, IT FEELS GOOD TO BE RESPONSIBLE

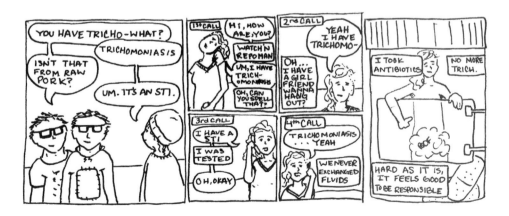

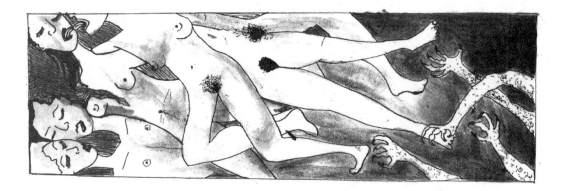

We felt the world changing around us, swelling together like a wave and lifting us up. We became adults in the age of *The L Word*, while we witnessed queer youth being bullied to the point of suicide. We watched Madonna make out with Britney Spears. We watch politicians arm wrestle over same-sex marriage laws while our friends throw punk shows to afford their healthcare and hormones and top surgery. We watch street harassment and police brutality everyday.

We are full of contradictions, but so is the world outside. We know that a different future is brewing, and we want to drink it in. We know that while we can only tell about our own lives, we are not alone. It took a lot of people to tell these stories. We promise not to let it end with us. After all, these are experiences, not answers.

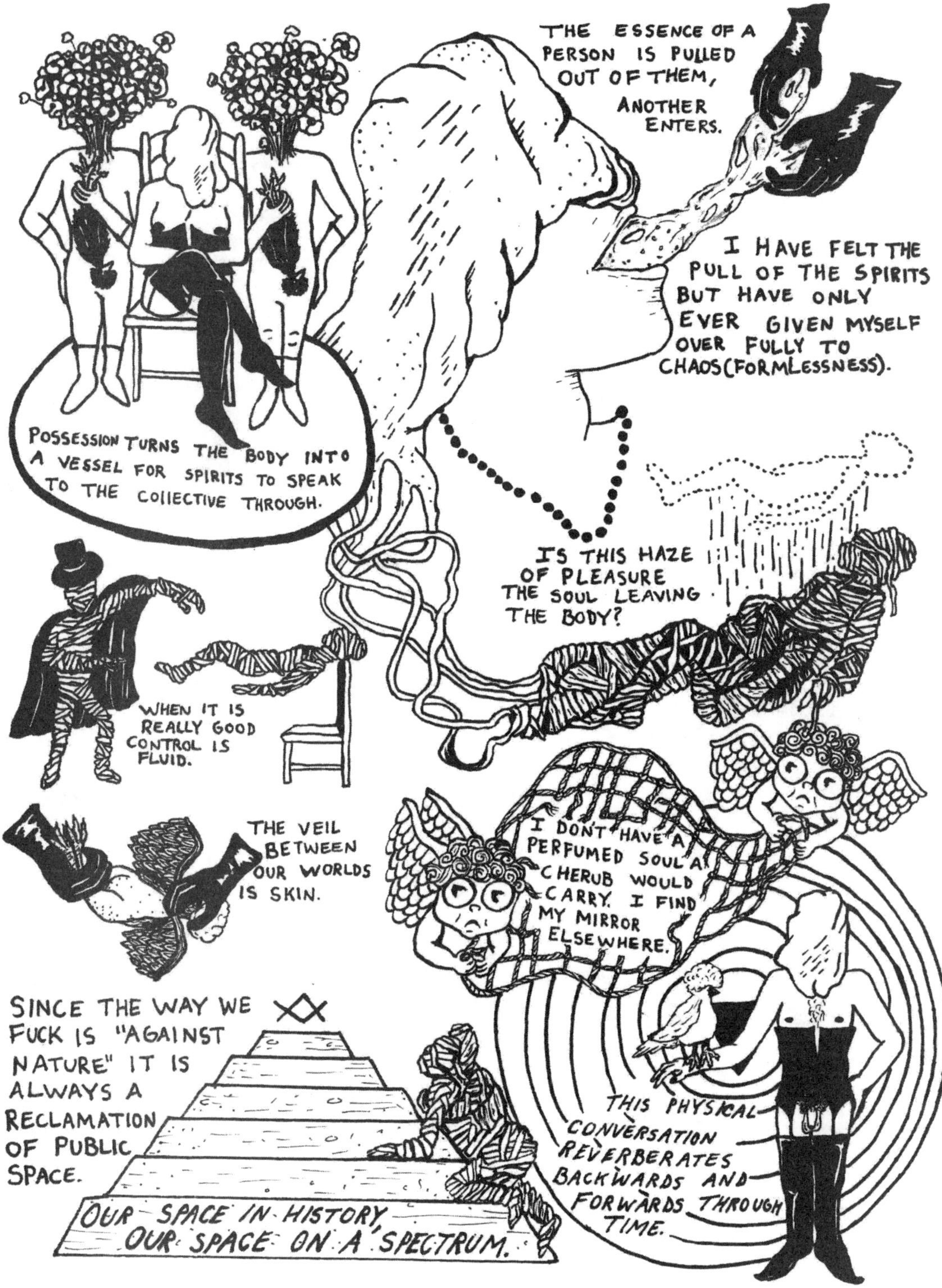

POSSESSION TURNS THE BODY INTO A VESSEL FOR SPIRITS TO SPEAK TO THE COLLECTIVE THROUGH.
THE ESSENCE OF A PERSON IS PULLED OUT OF THEM, ANOTHER ENTERS.
I HAVE FELT THE PULL OF THE SPIRITS BUT HAVE ONLY EVER GIVEN MYSELF OVER FULLY TO CHAOS(FORMLESSNESS).
IS THIS HAZE OF PLEASURE THE SOUL LEAVING THE BODY?
WHEN IT IS REALLY GOOD CONTROL IS FLUID.
THE VEIL BETWEEN OUR WORLDS IS SKIN.
I DON'T HAVE A PERFUMED SOUL A CHERUB WOULD CARRY. I FIND MY MIRROR ELSEWHERE.
SINCE THE WAY WE FUCK IS "AGAINST NATURE" IT IS ALWAYS A RECLAMATION OF PUBLIC SPACE.
OUR SPACE IN HISTORY, OUR SPACE ON A SPECTRUM.
THIS PHYSICAL CONVERSATION REVERBERATES BACKWARDS AND FORWARDS THROUGH TIME.

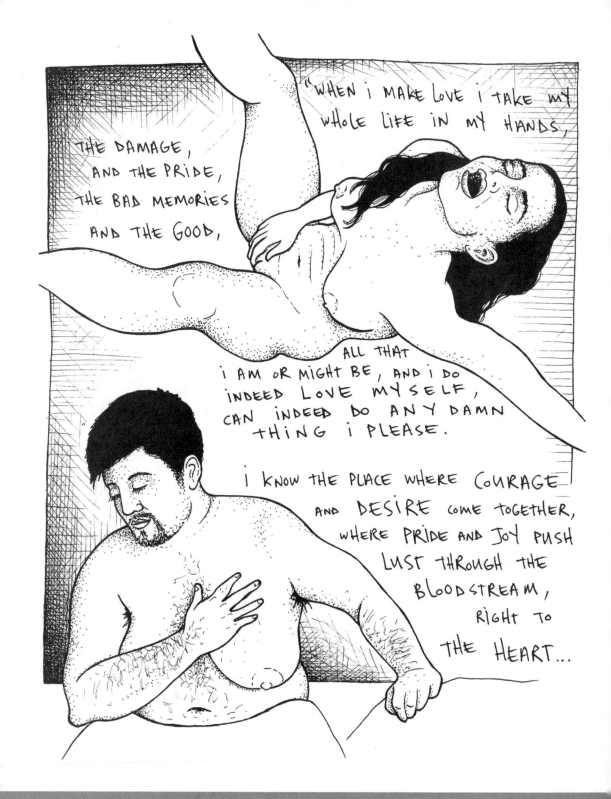

"WHEN I MAKE LOVE I TAKE MY WHOLE LIFE IN MY HANDS,

THE DAMAGE, AND THE PRIDE, THE BAD MEMORIES AND THE GOOD,

ALL THAT I AM OR MIGHT BE, AND I DO INDEED LOVE MYSELF, CAN INDEED DO ANY DAMN THING I PLEASE.

I KNOW THE PLACE WHERE COURAGE AND DESIRE COME TOGETHER, WHERE PRIDE AND JOY PUSH LUST THROUGH THE BLOODSTREAM, RIGHT TO THE HEART...

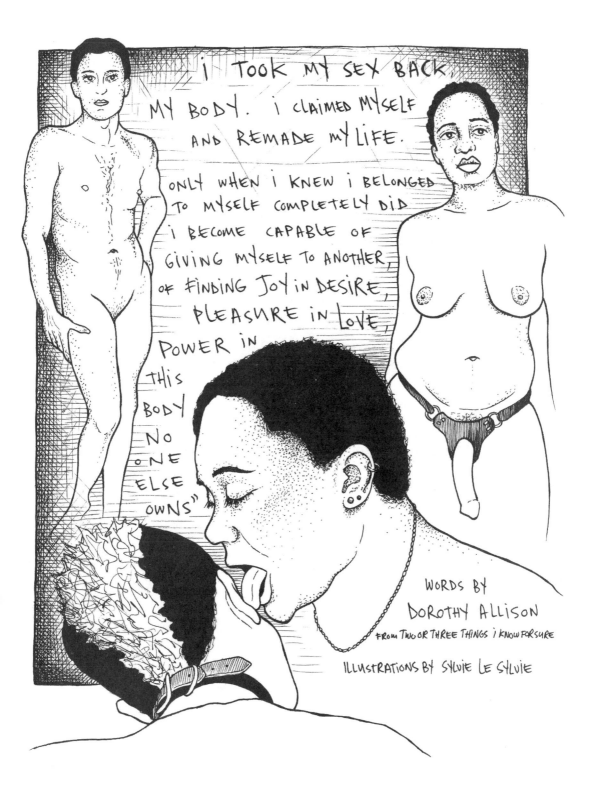

"i TOOK MY SEX BACK, MY BODY. i CLAIMED MYSELF AND REMADE MY LIFE.

ONLY WHEN i KNEW i BELONGED TO MYSELF COMPLETELY DID i BECOME CAPABLE OF GIVING MYSELF TO ANOTHER, OF FINDING JOY IN DESIRE, PLEASURE IN LOVE, POWER IN THIS BODY NO ONE ELSE OWNS"

WORDS BY DOROTHY ALLISON
FROM TWO OR THREE THINGS i KNOW FOR SURE

ILLUSTRATIONS BY SYLVIE LE SYLVIE

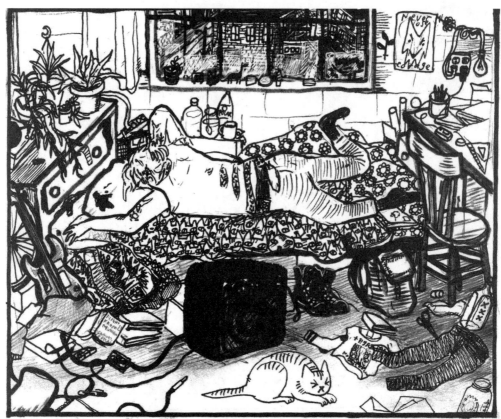

THE STORY OF A BLOSSOMING, PROGRESSIVE & SUCCESFUL QUEER MATURITY & ACTUALIZATION IS A STAGE SET FOR DISSAPOINTMENT. IT WON'T GET BETTER BECAUSE I WILL LIKELY ETERNALLY DEAL WITH SOME VERSION OF THE SAME SHIT WHICH UNDENIABLY SHAPES MY UNDERSTANDING OF MY BODY - AND MY ABILITY TO RELATE TO OTHERS. BUT I AM A QUEER ADULT AND THAT MEANS I CAN STAY UP TIL' 5 AM AND FUCK WITH MY CLOTHES ON AND PUT MY WHOLE HAND IN SOMEONE'S WARM BODY.

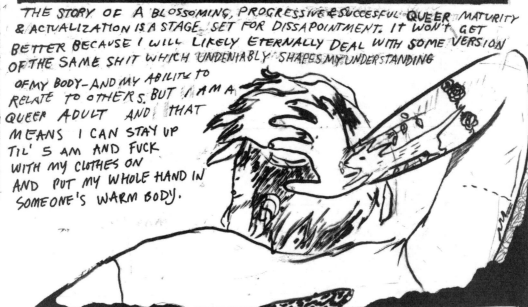

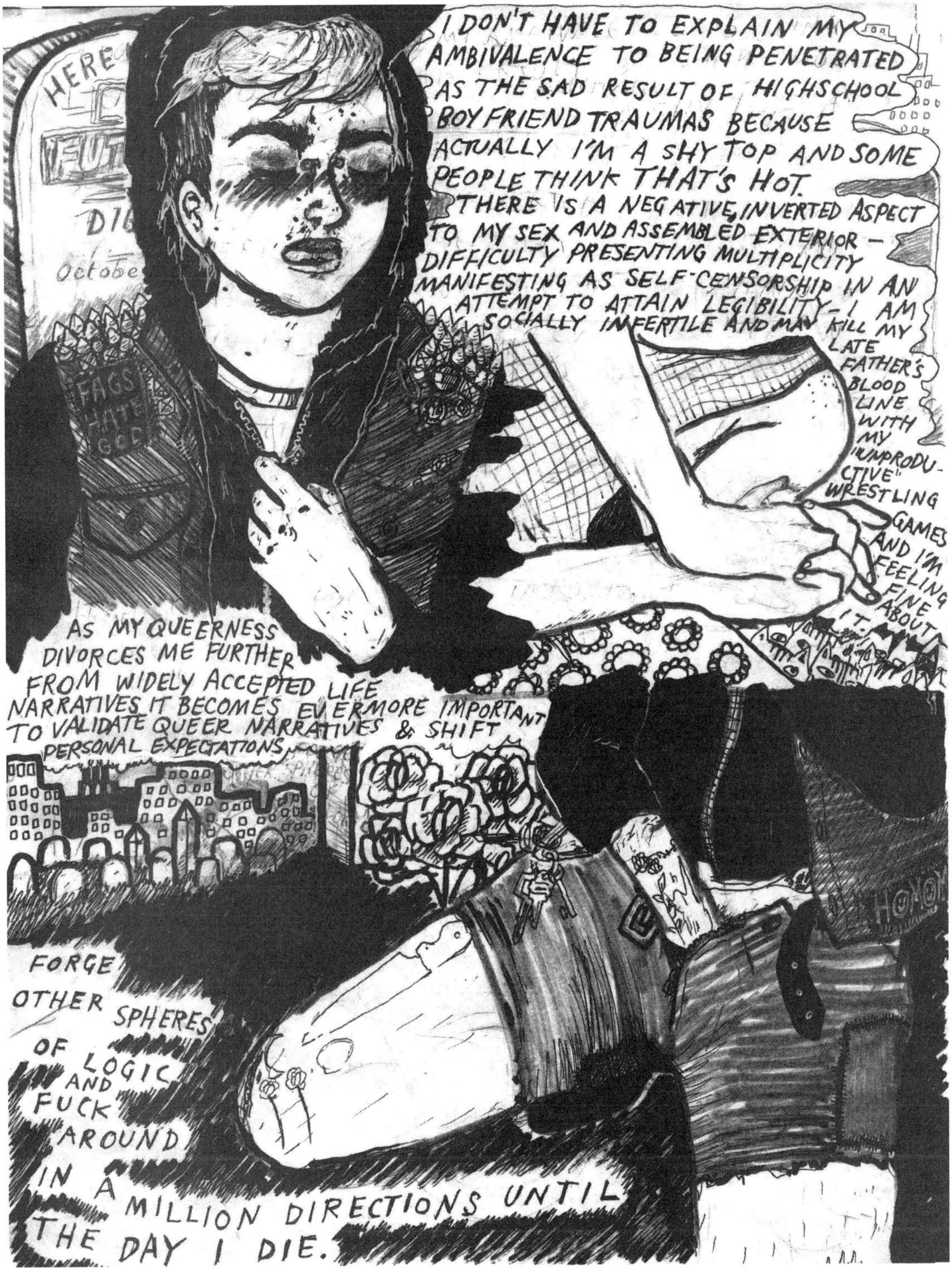
I DON'T HAVE TO EXPLAIN MY AMBIVALENCE TO BEING PENETRATED AS THE SAD RESULT OF HIGHSCHOOL BOY FRIEND TRAUMAS BECAUSE ACTUALLY I'M A SHY TOP AND SOME PEOPLE THINK THAT'S HOT.
THERE IS A NEGATIVE, INVERTED ASPECT TO MY SEX AND ASSEMBLED EXTERIOR — DIFFICULTY PRESENTING MULTIPLICITY MANIFESTING AS SELF-CENSORSHIP IN AN ATTEMPT TO ATTAIN LEGIBILITY - I AM SOCIALLY INFERTILE AND MAY KILL MY LATE FATHER'S BLOOD LINE WITH MY "UNPRODUCTIVE" WRESTLING GAMES AND I'M FEELING FINE ABOUT IT.
FAGS HATE GOD
AS MY QUEERNESS DIVORCES ME FURTHER FROM WIDELY ACCEPTED LIFE NARRATIVES IT BECOMES EVERMORE IMPORTANT TO VALIDATE QUEER NARRATIVES & SHIFT PERSONAL EXPECTATIONS,
FORGE OTHER SPHERES OF LOGIC AND FUCK AROUND IN A MILLION DIRECTIONS UNTIL THE DAY I DIE.

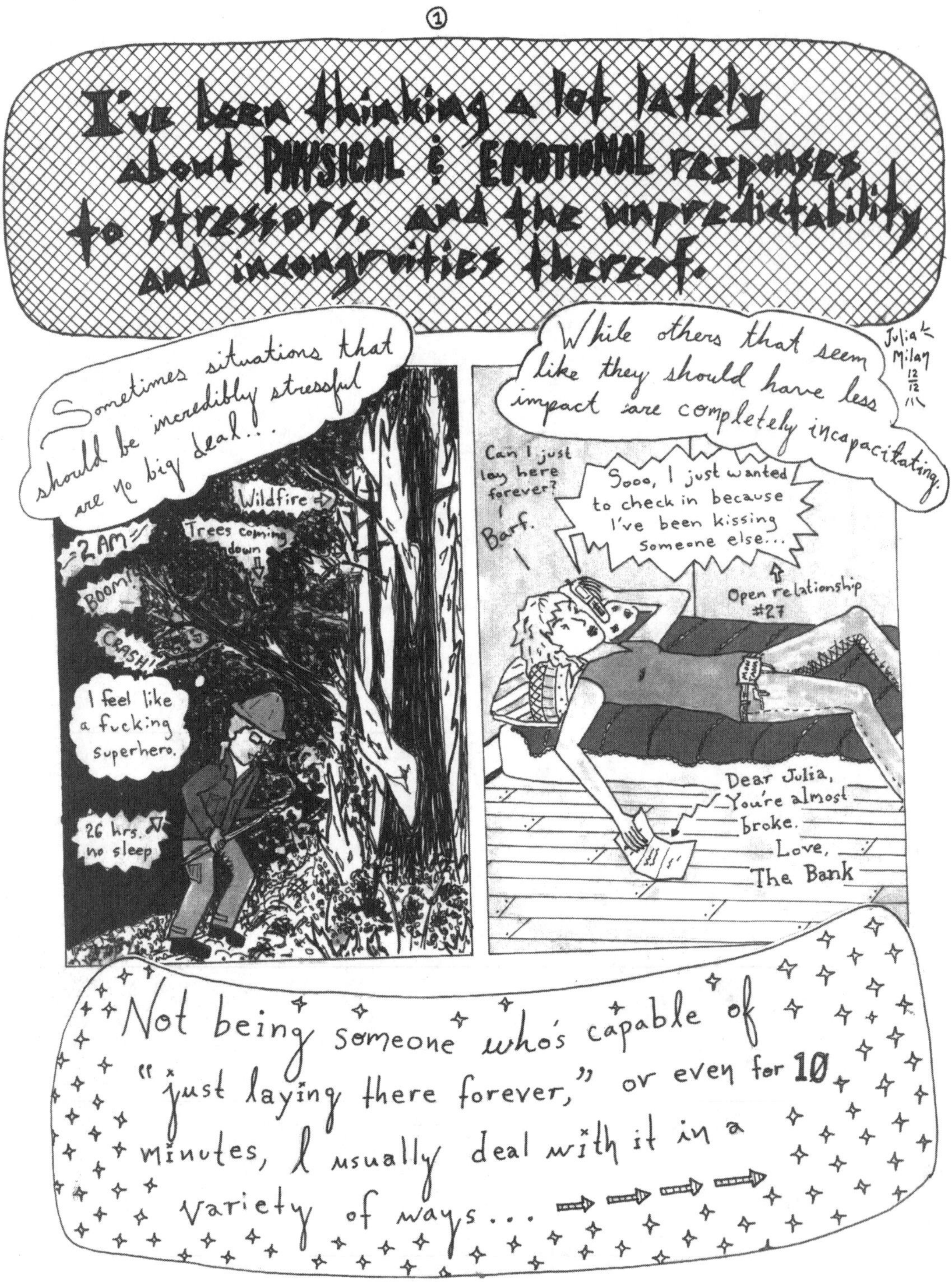

1
I've been thinking a lot lately about PHYSICAL & EMOTIONAL responses to stressors, and the unpredictability and incongruities thereof.
Sometimes situations that should be incredibly stressful are no big deal...
Wildfire
Trees coming down
2 AM
BOOM!
CRASH!
I feel like a fucking superhero.
26 hrs. no sleep
While others that seem like they should have less impact are completely incapacitating.
Julia Milan 12/12
Can I just lay here forever?
Barf.
Sooo, I just wanted to check in because I've been kissing someone else...
Open relationship #27
Dear Julia, You're almost broke. Love, The Bank
Not being someone who's capable of "just laying there forever," or even for 10 minutes, I usually deal with it in a variety of ways...

2
SOME OF THEM ARE PRODUCTIVE
Tea
Herbs
Excercise
Spelling
Why Cats Paint
Walking with Crystals
The Endurance
Books
eating well
perfection!
makin' mixtapes
Two unopened gallons of olive oil and a window scraper dressed like a little santa!?!
Rekindling love with The Garbage
OTHERS, NOT SO MUCH
Booze + Cigs
What did you do today?
Nothing
No, really
Well, it might as well have been nothing.
general Apathy
Can we just talk about why you're being a spineless urchin who keeps hurting my feelings?
Can we please not right now?
No we're going to talk now. I have 2 hours.
Okay.
Always weirdly matching...
Where'd you say you were from again?
Kiss
Kiss
Not important.
Random Hookups *
Running the fuck Away
Tactless Over-processing
* Not that random hookups are always bad, just usually not so healthy for me.

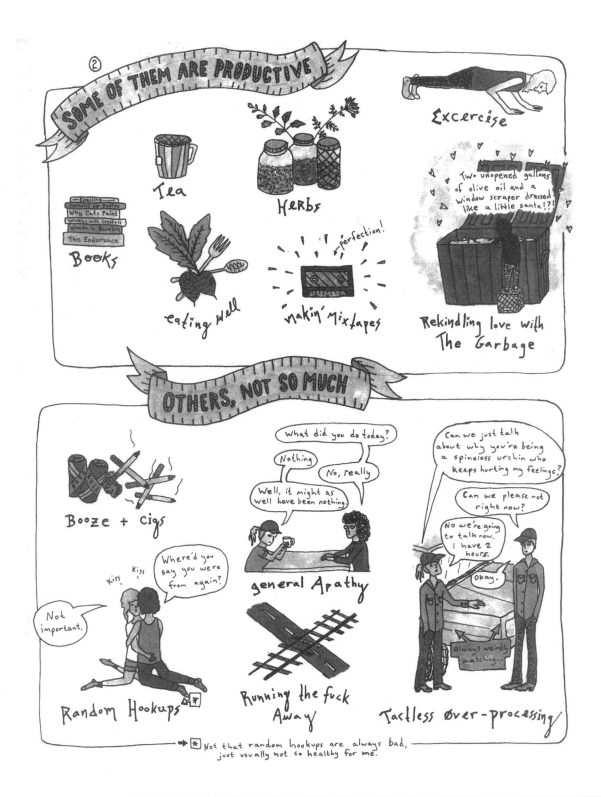

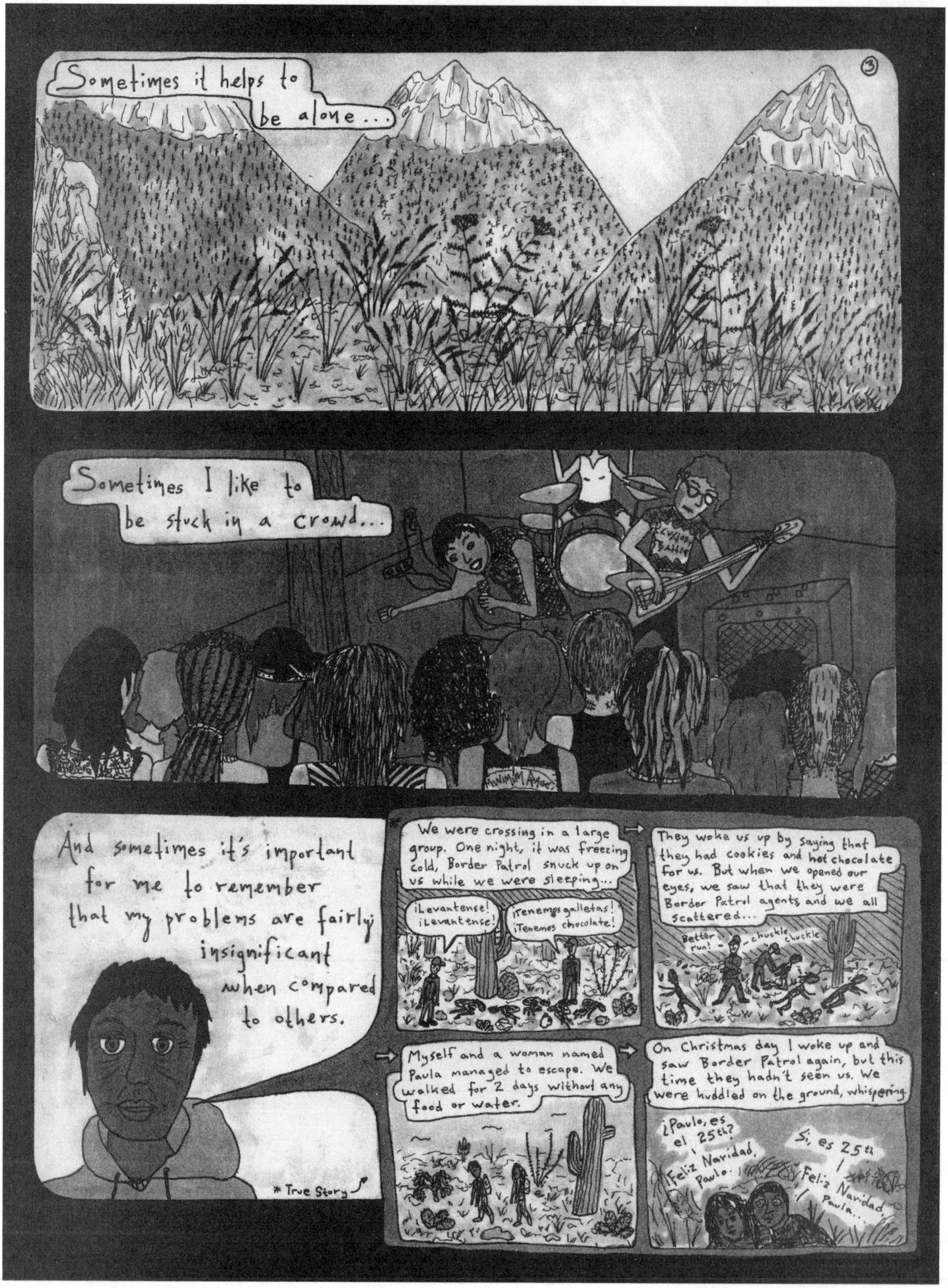

3
Sometimes it helps to be alone...
Sometimes I like to be stuck in a crowd...
And sometimes it's important for me to remember that my problems are fairly insignificant when compared to others.
* True Story
We were crossing in a large group. One night, it was freezing cold, Border Patrol snuck up on us while we were sleeping...
¡Levantense! ¡Levantense!
¡Tenemos galletas! ¡Tenemos chocolate!
They woke us up by saying that they had cookies and hot chocolate for us. But when we opened our eyes, we saw that they were Border Patrol agents and we all scattered...
Better run!
chuckle chuckle
Myself and a woman named Paula managed to escape. We walked for 2 days without any food or water.
On Christmas day I woke up and saw Border Patrol again, but this time they hadn't seen us. We were huddled on the ground, whispering.
¿Paulo, es el 25th?
Feliz Navidad, Paulo.
Si, es 25th
Feliz Navidad, Paula...

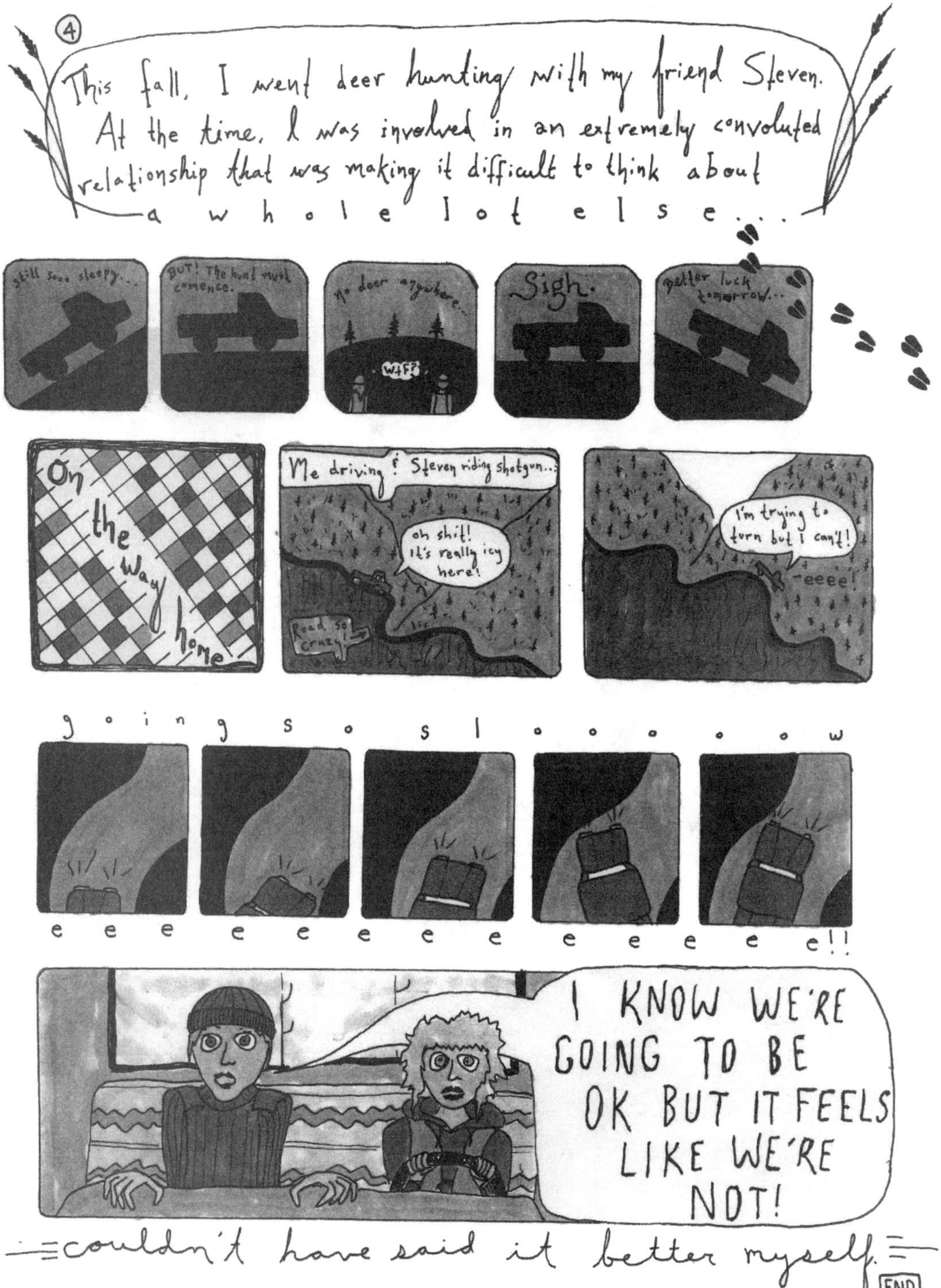
4
This fall, I went deer hunting with my friend Steven. At the time, I was involved in an extremely convoluted relationship that was making it difficult to think about a whole lot else...
still sooo sleepy...
BUT! The hunt must comence.
no deer anywhere...
WTF?
Sigh.
better luck tomorrow...
On the way home
Me driving & Steven riding shotgun...
oh shit! it's really icy here!
Road so crazy!
I'm trying to turn but I can't!
eeee!
going so sloooow
eeeeeeeeeeeee!!
I KNOW WE'RE GOING TO BE OK BUT IT FEELS LIKE WE'RE NOT!
couldn't have said it better myself.
END

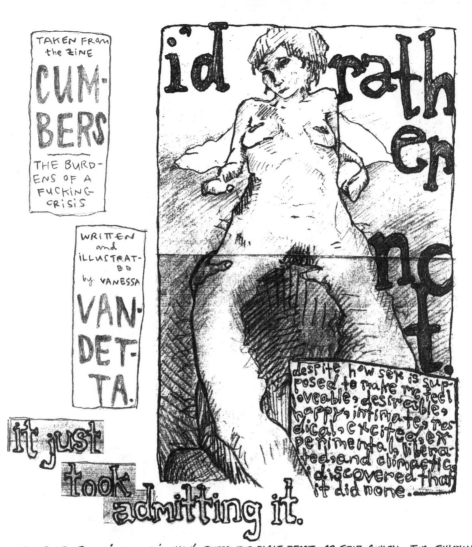

TAKEN FROM the ZINE

CUMBERS

THE BURDENS OF A FUCKING CRISIS

WRITTEN and ILLUSTRATED by VANESSA VANDETTA.

id rather not.

despite how sex is supposed to make me feel loveable, desirable, happy, intimate, radical, excited, experimental, liberated, and climactic, i discovered that it did none.

it just took admitting it.

AND THAT IT WASN'T BECAUSE i HADN'T FUCKED THE RIGHT PEOPLE, OR FELT GUILTY FOR ENJOYING SEXUAL PLEASURES OR BECAUSE i HAD RELIGIOUS CONFLICTS, OR WAS INSECURE ABOUT MY BODY AND MY SEXUAL "PERFORMANCE" BEING HOT ENOUGH. THAT IT WASN'T BECAUSE I WAS REPRESSING TABOOED LONGINGS, OR BECAUSE I ASSOCIATED SEX WITH VIOLATION AS A RESULT OF HAVING BEEN SEXUALLY ASSAULTED BEFORE. THAT IT WASN'T BECAUSE I WAS EITHER TOO STRAIGHT OR TOO GAY THAT I LATCHED SEXUAL IMPULSE AND ATTRACTION TOWARDS ANY PEOPLE IN PARTICULAR, BUT THAT i OPERATED ON A DIFFERENT LEVEL OF INTEREST IN ALL THINGS SEXUAL, ALL TOGETHER, THAN WHAT I HAD BEEN REQUIRING OF MYSELF. ————————————————————→ I HAVE, FOR WHATEVER THE REASONS, LIMITED INSIGHT INTO THE REASONS FOR WHY SEX AND SEXUALLY CHARGED INTERACTIONS FALL SHORT OF DELIVERING ME TO ANY OF THE HEIGHTENED STATES OF EXISTENCE I'VE HAD PRESENTED TO ME AS POSSIBILITIES. OF COURSE COMPLICATING THIS PROCESS OF SELF-REFLECTION & ANALYSIS FURTHER IS THE FACT THAT I REALLY ONLY HAVE OTHER OTHER PEOPLE'S PROJECTIONS OF THEIR EXPERIENCES TO GO FROM AS A BASIS OF COMPARISON, PEOPLE WHO, IF THEY ARE ANYTHING LIKE ME, MIGHT HAVE A DIFFICULT TIME ADMITTING IF & WHEN THEIR SEXUAL EXPERIENCES—THAT IS, THEIR EXPERIENCES OF SEXUAL SITUATIONS—FAIL TO CORRESPOND WITH SIMILAR IMAGES OF COMFORTABILITY & EXALTATION AS THOSE WHICH I HAD BECOME USED TO REGARDING AS EVIDENCE OF MY FLAWED COMPOSITION AS A FEELING BEING

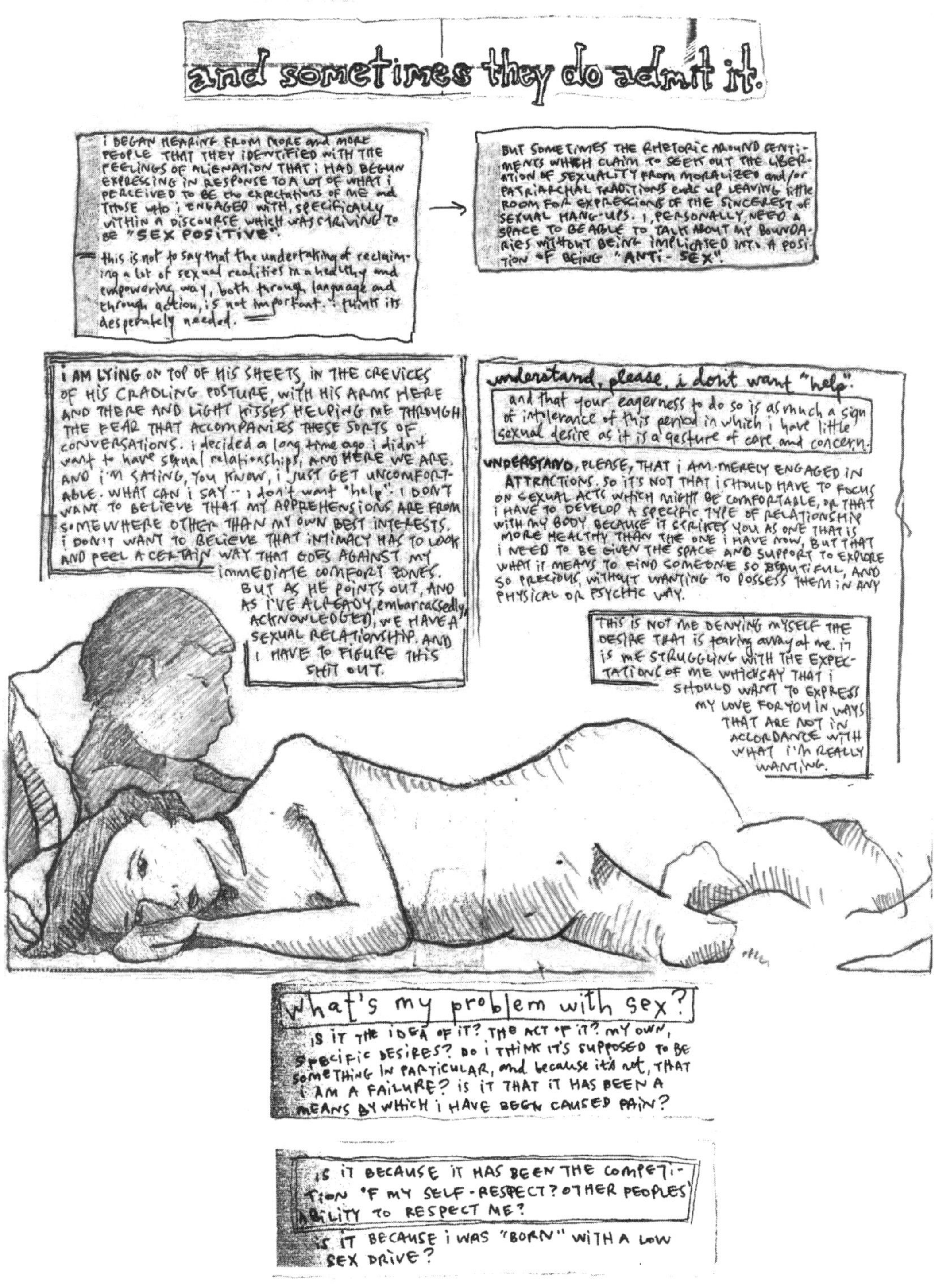
and sometimes they do admit it.
i BEGAN HEARING FROM MORE and MORE PEOPLE THAT THEY iDENTiFIED WiTH THE FEELINGS OF ALiENATiON THAT i HAD BEGUN EXPRESSING iN RESPONSE TO A LOT OF WHAT i PERCEIVED TO BE the expectations of ME and THOSE WHO i ENGAGED WiTH, SPECiFiCALLY WiTHIN A DiSCOURSE WHiCH WAS STRiViNG TO BE "SEX POSiTiVE".
this is not to say that the undertaking of reclaiming a lot of sexual realities in a healthy and empowering way, both through language and through action, is not important. i think its desperately needed.
BUT SOMETiMES THE RHETORiC AROUND SENTiMENTS WHICH CLAiM TO SEEK OUT THE LiBERATiON OF SEXUALiTY FROM MORALiZED and/or PATRiARCHAL TRADiTiONS ends up LEAViNG little ROOM FOR EXPRESSiONS OF THE SiNCEREST of SEXUAL HANG-UPS. i, PERSONALLY, NEED A SPACE TO BE ABLE TO TALK ABOUT MY BOUNDARiES WiTHOUT BEiNG iMPLiCATED iNTO A POSiTiON OF BEiNG "ANTi-SEX".
i AM LYiNG ON TOP OF HiS SHEETS, iN THE CREViCES OF HiS CRADLiNG POSTURE, WiTH HiS ARMS HERE AND THERE AND LiGHT KiSSES HELPiNG ME THROUGH THE FEAR THAT ACCOMPANiES THESE SORTS OF CONVERSATiONS. i decided a long time ago i didn't want to have sexual relationships, AND HERE WE ARE. AND i'M SAYiNG, YOU KNOW, i JUST GET UNCOMFORTABLE. WHAT CAN i SAY-- i don't want "help". i DON'T WANT TO BELiEVE THAT MY APPREHENSiONS ARE FROM SOMEWHERE OTHER THAN MY OWN BEST iNTERESTS. i DON'T WANT TO BELiEVE THAT iNTiMACY HAS TO LOOK AND FEEL A CERTAiN WAY THAT GOES AGAiNST MY iMMEDiATE COMFORT ZONES.
BUT AS HE POiNTS OUT, AND AS i'VE ALREADY, embarrassedly, ACKNOWLEDGED, WE HAVE A SEXUAL RELATiONSHiP. AND i HAVE TO FiGURE THiS SHiT OUT.
understand, please, i don't want "help".
and that your eagerness to do so is as much a sign of intolerance of this period in which i have little sexual desire as it is a gesture of care and concern.
UNDERSTAND, PLEASE, THAT i AM MERELY ENGAGED iN ATTRACTiONS. SO iT'S NOT THAT i SHOULD HAVE TO FOCUS ON SEXUAL ACTS WHiCH MiGHT BE COMFORTABLE, OR THAT i HAVE TO DEVELOP A SPECiFiC TYPE OF RELATiONSHiP WiTH MY BODY BECAUSE iT STRiKES YOU AS ONE THAT iS MORE HEALTHY THAN THE ONE i HAVE NOW, BUT THAT i NEED TO BE GiVEN THE SPACE AND SUPPORT TO EXPLORE WHAT iT MEANS TO FiND SOMEONE SO BEAUTiFUL, AND SO PRECiOUS, WiTHOUT WANTiNG TO POSSESS THEM iN ANY PHYSiCAL OR PSYCHiC WAY.
THiS iS NOT ME DENYiNG MYSELF THE DESiRE THAT iS tearing away at me. iT iS ME STRUGGLiNG WiTH THE EXPECTATiONS OF ME WHiCH SAY THAT i SHOULD WANT TO EXPRESS MY LOVE FOR YOU iN WAYS THAT ARE NOT iN ACCORDANCE WiTH WHAT i'M REALLY WANTiNG.
what's my problem with sex?
iS iT THE iDEA OF iT? THE ACT OF iT? MY OWN, SPECiFiC DESiRES? DO i THiNK iT'S SUPPOSED TO BE SOMETHiNG iN PARTiCULAR, and because it's not, THAT i AM A FAiLURE? iS iT THAT iT HAS BEEN A MEANS BY WHiCH i HAVE BEEN CAUSED PAiN?
iS iT BECAUSE iT HAS BEEN THE COMPETiTiON OF MY SELF-RESPECT? OTHER PEOPLES' ABiLiTY TO RESPECT ME?
iS iT BECAUSE i WAS "BORN" WiTH A LOW SEX DRiVE?

OR BECAUSE i FEEL CHEAPENED BY BECOMING THE OBJECT OF SOMEONE'S FANCY? BECAUSE i FEEL INCAPABLE OF TURNING SOMEONE ELSE INTO THE OBJECT OF MY OWN FANCY?

IS iT BECAUSE i HAVE HAD TOO MANY "BAD" LOVERS?

OR LOVERS WHO DIDN'T GIVE ME POSITIVE REINFORCEMENT ABOUT MY OWN SEXUAL BEHAVIOUR?

and WHY SEX?

WHY SUCH A COMMON FORM OF VIOLENCE? WHY SO OFTEN TALKED ABOUT? WHY SO SCARY? WHY SO FUN? WHY DOES iT CAUSE SO MUCH JEALOUSY? WHY IS iT USED TO VALIDATE ONE'S WORTH? WHY IS iT THE THING WE CHOOSE TO FOCUS ON AND NARROW DOWN WHEN EVERY ASPECT OF OURSELVES IS AS COMPLICATED AND UNIQUE AS THAT OF OUR SEXUALITIES?

SEX ACTS, UP TILL A POINT, i KNOW INVOLVE MY FEELINGS ABOUT AND/OR ATTRACTION TO THE OTHER PERSON. BUT AT SOME point EITHER ON THE BODY OR IN THE HEAT, iT CAN START TO FEEL LIKE WE ARE JUST TRYING TO GET THE OTHER OFF. i DON'T WANT TO HAVE TO WORRY ABOUT SATISFYING ANY ONE, NOT THEM, ME.

AND i DON'T WANT TO OR HAVE TO USE THEM TO GET OFF.... I DON'T FEEL COMFORTABLE WITH THE MENTAL TRANSITIONS, PLAYING SEXY, TURNING SOMEONE ELSE INTO "SEX OBJECT" -- YET AS MUCH AS i KNOW THAT THAT IS NOT THE ONLY WAY OF UNDERSTANDING THE EXPERIENCE, I CAN'T HELP BUT SEE ALL OF WHAT IS HAPPENING AS JUST THAT.

THIS AWARENESS BEGAN WHILE i WAS STILL IN A VERY INTENSE ROMANTIC RELATIONSHIP WITH A PERSON WHO i WAS STILL VERY SEXUALLY ATTRACTED TO BUT WITH WHOM i FELT SEX HAD BECOME AN EXTREMELY DIVISIVE ISSUE. AT ONE POINT, i BEGAN TO REALISE HOW MUCH SECURITY i HAD INVESTED IN THE PEOPLE i HAD GOTTEN BUSY WITH ON THE BASIS THAT i SHARED WITH THEM SOMETHING i FELT VERY UN- COMFORTABLE WITH IN THE FIRST PLACE AND THAT MADE ME FEEL EVEN WORSE FOR HOW MUCH iT RESEMBLED BEING

possessed! -OR- tied down!

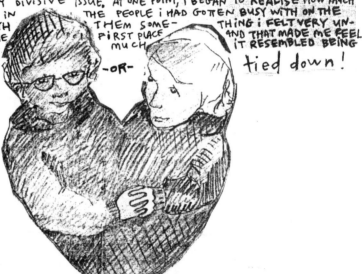

i WISH THAT A WILL WERE ALL THAT WAS NECESSARY TO RID MYSELF OF THE AWFUL SUSPICION THAT MUTUAL SUPPORT IS IMPOSSIBLE WITHOUT MUTUAL POSSESSION, THAT FRIENDSHIP CAN NEVER VALIDATE INTIMACY THE WAY THAT SEX PRETENDS TO, THAT SEX IS THE PROOF OF EXCEPTIONALITY, THAT EXCEPTIONALITY IS WHAT QUALIFIES INTIMACY, AND THAT THE TASK OF DEVELOPING CONFIDENCE IN A BETTER SYSTEM INVOLVES TAKING RISKS THAT FEW PEOPLE WOULD BE WILLING TO TAKE.

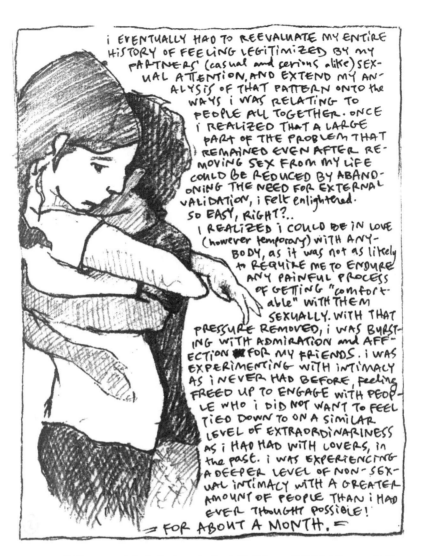

i EVENTUALLY HAD TO REEVALUATE MY ENTIRE HISTORY OF FEELING LEGITIMIZED BY MY PARTNERS' (casual and serious alike) SEXUAL ATTENTION, AND EXTEND MY ANALYSIS OF THAT PATTERN ONTO the WAYS i WAS RELATING TO PEOPLE ALL TOGETHER. ONCE i REALIZED THAT A LARGE PART OF THE PROBLEM THAT REMAINED EVEN AFTER REMOVING SEX FROM MY LIFE COULD BE REDUCED BY ABANDONING THE NEED FOR EXTERNAL VALIDATION, i FELT enlightened. SO EASY, RIGHT?..

I REALIZED i COULD BE IN LOVE (however temporary) WITH ANYBODY, AS it WAS NOT AS likely to REQUIRE ME TO ENDURE ANY PAINFUL PROCESS OF GETTING "comfortable" WITH THEM SEXUALLY. WITH THAT PRESSURE REMOVED, i WAS BURSTING WITH ADMIRATION and AFFECTION ✖ FOR MY FRIENDS. i WAS EXPERIMENTING WITH INTIMACY AS i NEVER HAD BEFORE, feeling FREED UP TO ENGAGE WITH PEOPLE WHO i DID NOT WANT TO FEEL TIED DOWN TO ON A SIMILAR LEVEL OF EXTRAORDINARINESS AS i HAD HAD WITH LOVERS, in the past. i WAS EXPERIENCING A DEEPER LEVEL OF NON-SEXUAL INTIMACY WITH A GREATER AMOUNT OF PEOPLE THAN i HAD EVER THOUGHT POSSIBLE!

⟹ FOR ABOUT A MONTH. ⟸

SO WHAT BEGAN AS SOMETHING THAT i PERCEIVED TO BE AN ISOLATED ISSUE OF ME HAVING TOO MANY SEXUAL HANG-UPS TO CONTINUE TO HAVE SEXUAL RELATIONSHIPS, HAS SLOWLY DEVELOPED INTO A MONUMENTAL CHANGE IN THE WAY i AM ABLE TO ENGAGE WITH OTHER PEOPLE AND RELATIONSHIPS IN GENERAL. i GUESS this DEVELOPMENT HAS HELPED TO INFORM ME ABOUT A LOT OF THE WAYS THAT MY ORIGINAL FEELINGS ABOUT SEX BEING UNCOMFORTABLE FOR ME WERE PARTIALLY BECAUSE OF ISSUES I HAVE, INTRAPERSONALLY, AROUND POWER and POSSESSION. MOREOVER, iT HAS EXPOSED ME TO THE FACT THAT MY EXPERIENCE OF SEXUAL SITUATIONS IS NOT JUST AN ARBITRARY, PHYSICAL MANIFESTATION OF DISCOMFORT THAT STEMS FROM SOMEWHERE UNRELATED; iT IS AS MUCH SOCIAL AS iT IS PERSONAL.

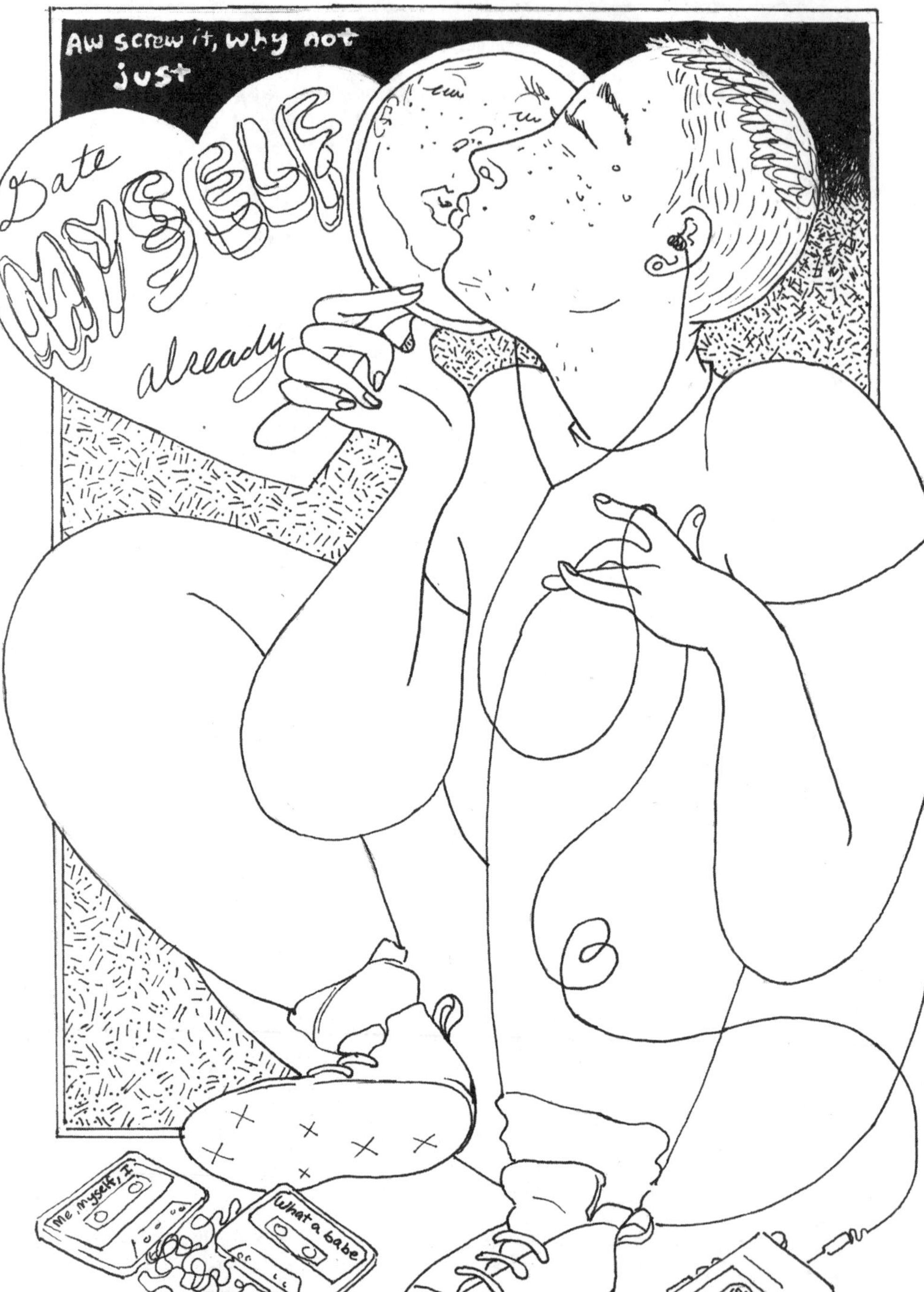
Aw screw it, why not just
Date
MYSELF
already
Me, myself, I
What a babe

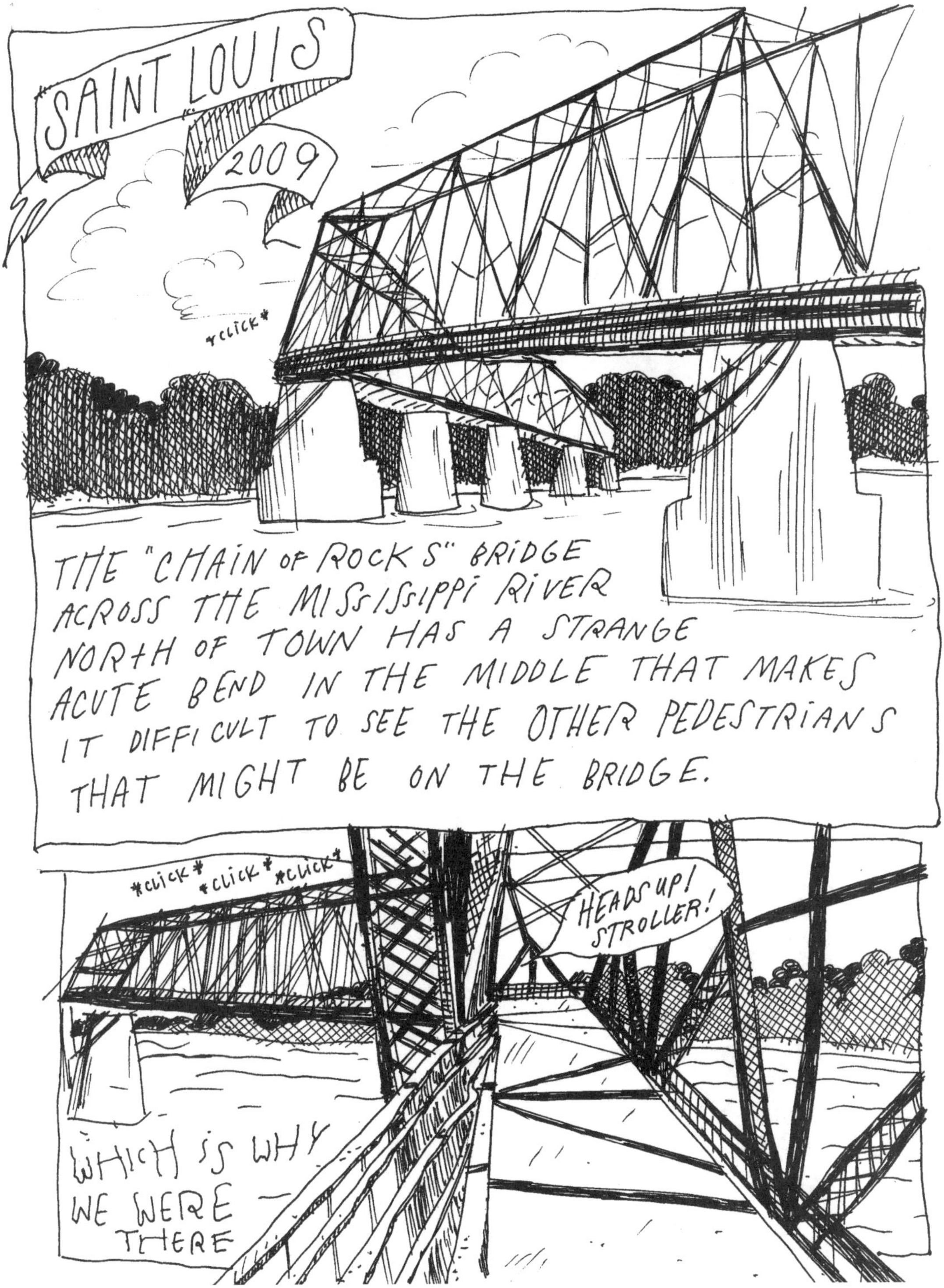
SAINT LOUIS
2009
CLICK
THE "CHAIN OF ROCKS" BRIDGE ACROSS THE MISSISSIPPI RIVER NORTH OF TOWN HAS A STRANGE ACUTE BEND IN THE MIDDLE THAT MAKES IT DIFFICULT TO SEE THE OTHER PEDESTRIANS THAT MIGHT BE ON THE BRIDGE.
CLICK *CLICK* *CLICK*
HEADS UP! STROLLER!
WHICH IS WHY WE WERE THERE

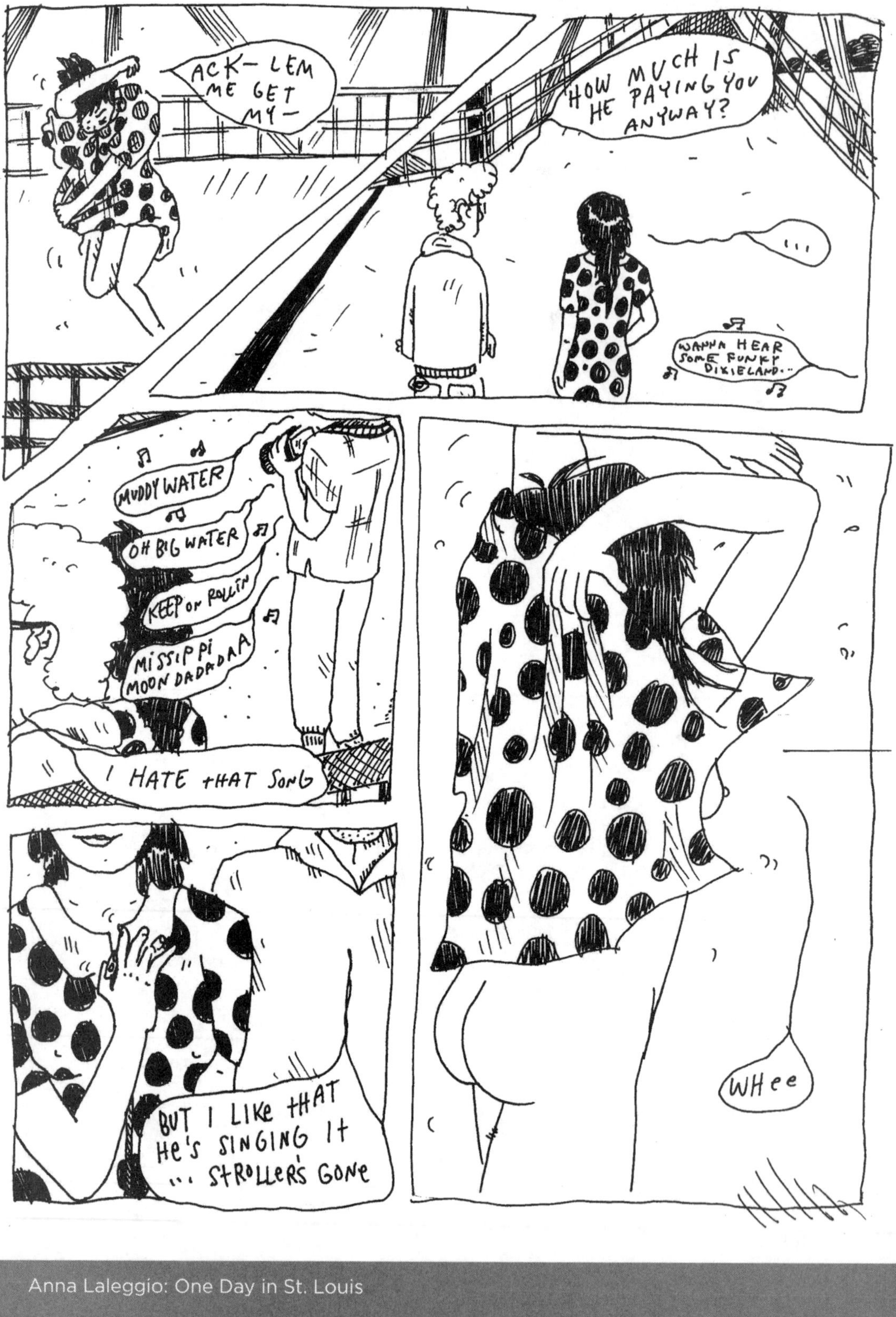
ACK— LEM ME GET MY—
HOW MUCH IS HE PAYING YOU ANYWAY?
...
WANNA HEAR SOME FUNKY DIXIELAND...
MUDDY WATER
OH BIG WATER
KEEP ON ROLLIN
MISSIPPI MOON DADADAA
I HATE THAT SONG
WHee
BUT I LIKE THAT He's SINGING It ... STROLLER'S GONE

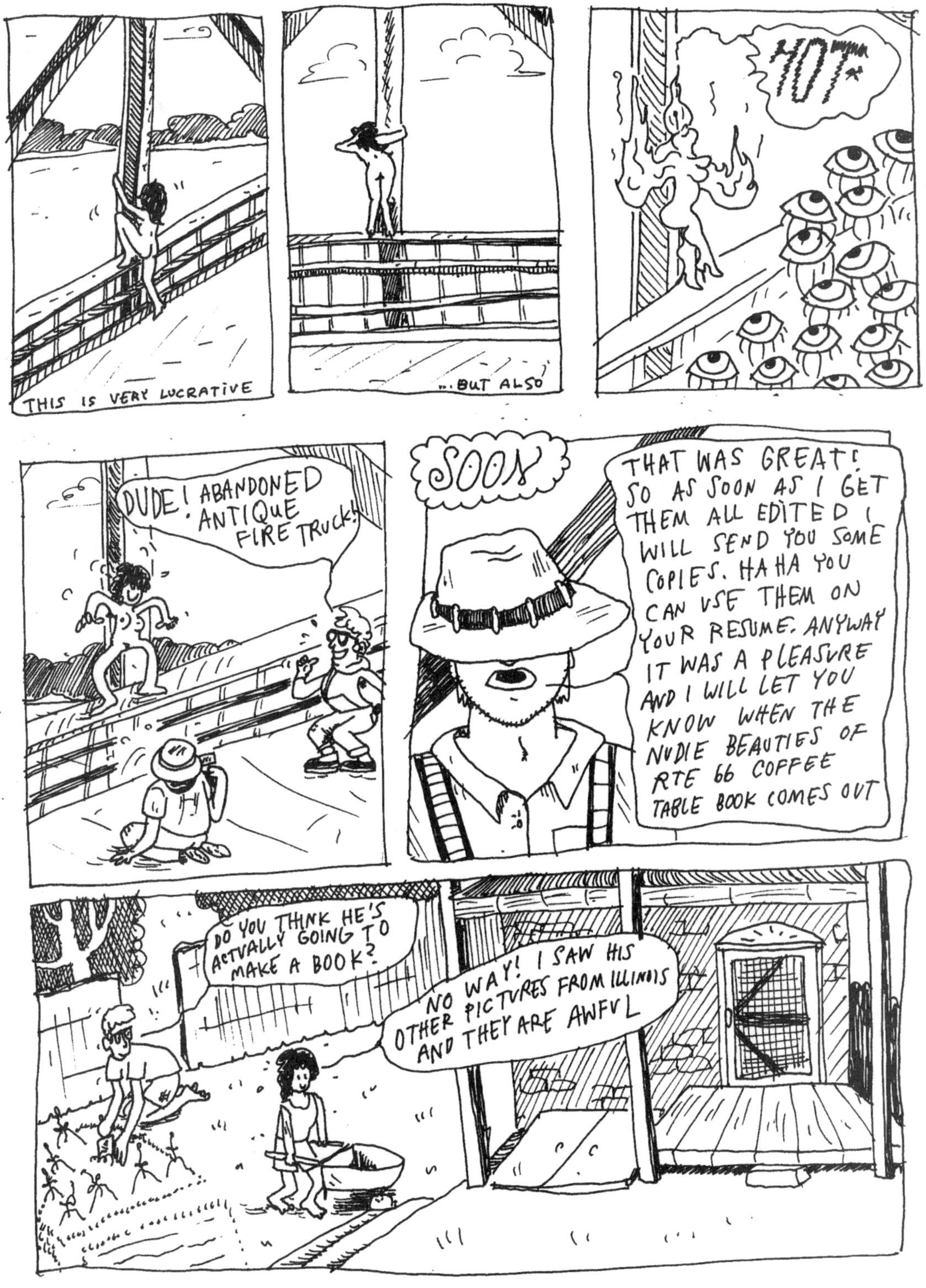
THIS IS VERY LUCRATIVE
...BUT ALSO
HOT*
DUDE! ABANDONED ANTIQUE FIRE TRUCK!
SOON
THAT WAS GREAT! SO AS SOON AS I GET THEM ALL EDITED I WILL SEND YOU SOME COPIES. HA HA YOU CAN USE THEM ON YOUR RESUME. ANYWAY IT WAS A PLEASURE AND I WILL LET YOU KNOW WHEN THE NUDIE BEAUTIES OF RTE 66 COFFEE TABLE BOOK COMES OUT
DO YOU THINK HE'S ACTUALLY GOING TO MAKE A BOOK?
NO WAY! I SAW HIS OTHER PICTURES FROM ILLINOIS AND THEY ARE AWFUL

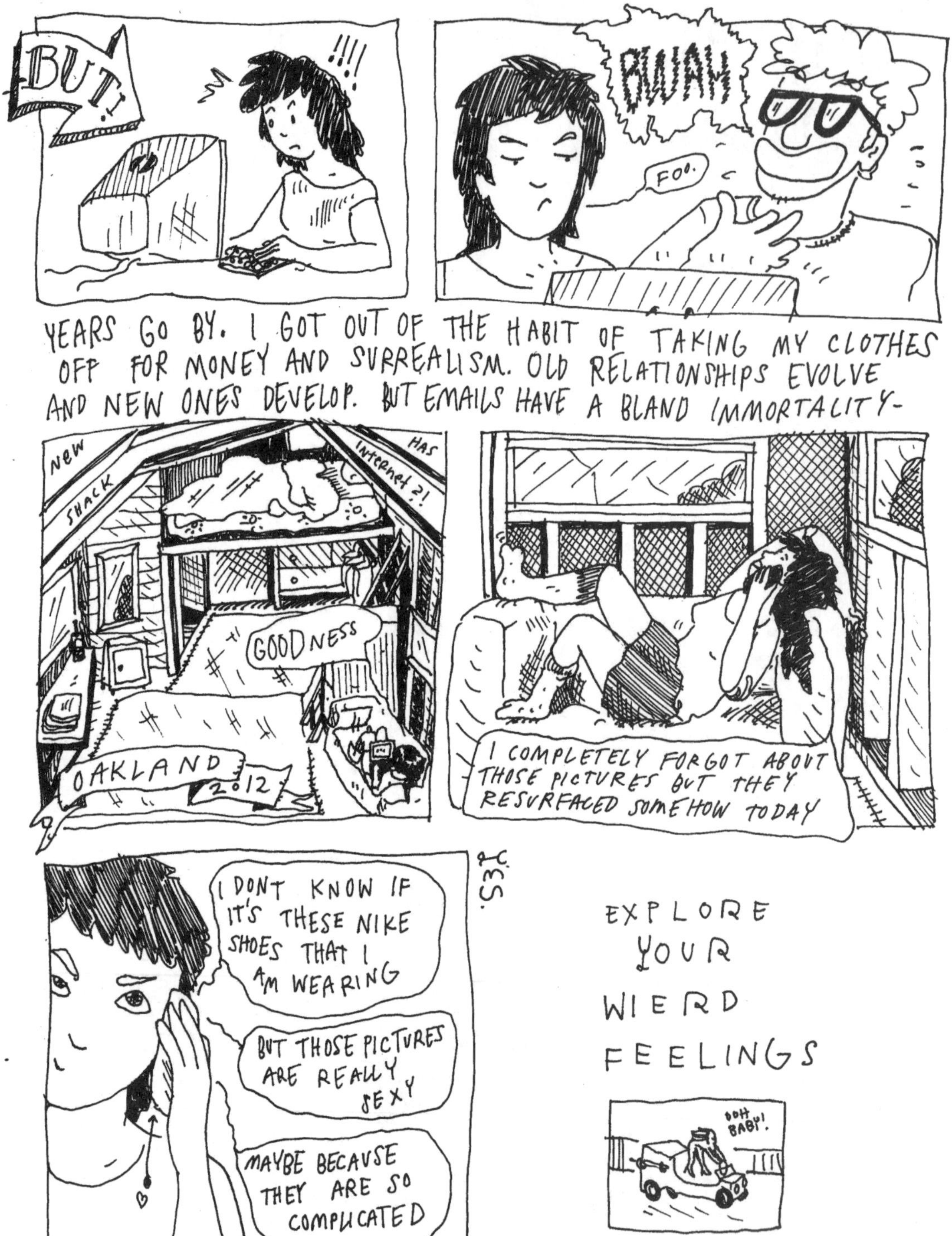
BUT!
!!!!
BWAH
FOO.
YEARS GO BY. I GOT OUT OF THE HABIT OF TAKING MY CLOTHES OFF FOR MONEY AND SURREALISM. OLD RELATIONSHIPS EVOLVE AND NEW ONES DEVELOP. BUT EMAILS HAVE A BLAND IMMORTALITY-
NEW SHACK
HAS INTERNET?!
GOODNESS
OAKLAND 2012
I COMPLETELY FORGOT ABOUT THOSE PICTURES BUT THEY RESURFACED SOMEHOW TODAY
I DONT KNOW IF IT'S THESE NIKE SHOES THAT I AM WEARING
BUT THOSE PICTURES ARE REALLY SEXY
MAYBE BECAUSE THEY ARE SO COMPLICATED
EXPLORE YOUR WIERD FEELINGS
OOH BABY!

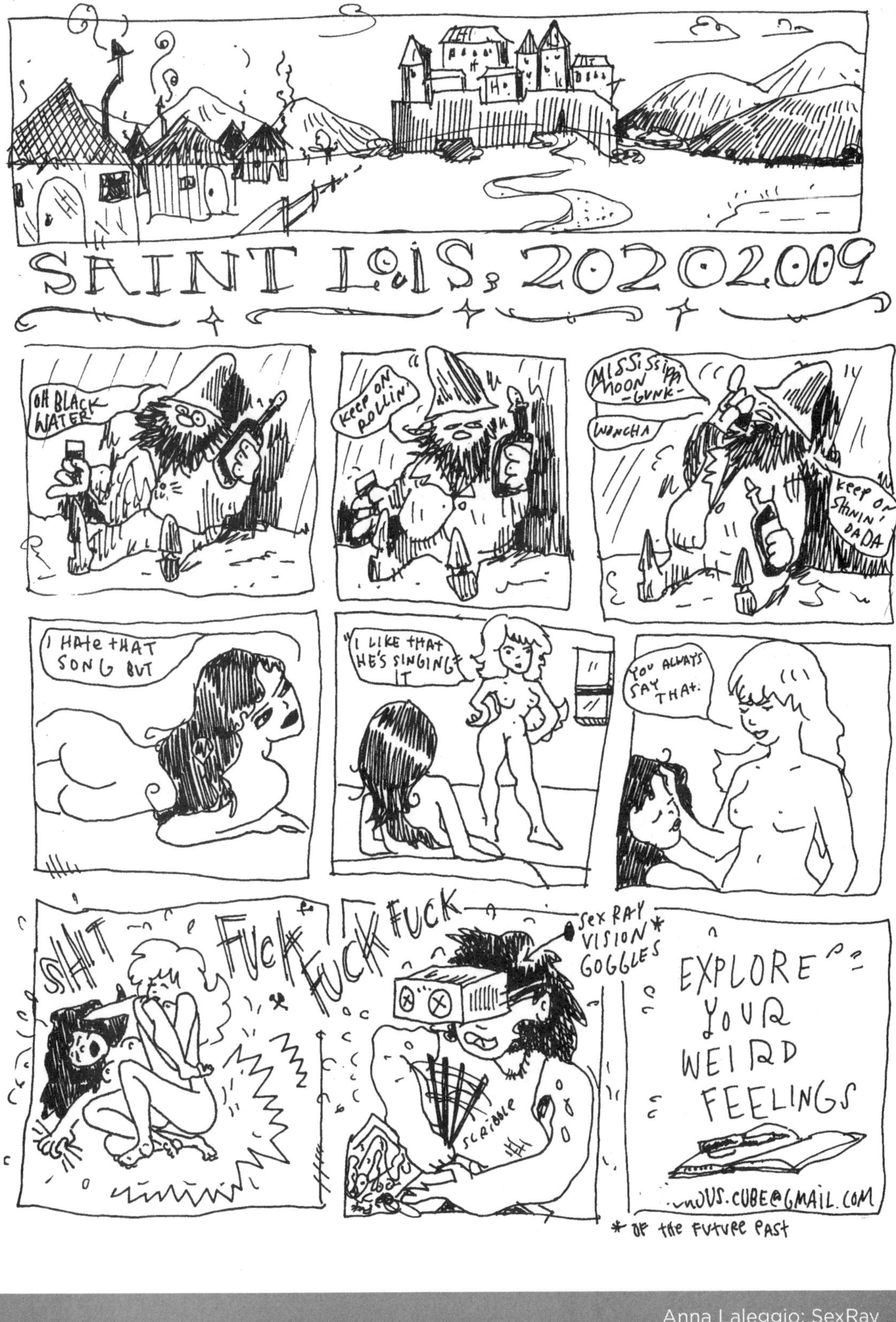
SAINT LOUIS, 2020 2009
OH BLACK WATER
KEEP ON ROLLIN'
MISSISSIPPI MOON -GUNK-
WONCHA
KEEP ON SHININ' DADA
I HATE THAT SONG BUT
I LIKE THAT HE'S SINGING IT
YOU ALWAYS SAY THAT.
SHIT
FUCK
FUCK FUCK
SEX RAY VISION* GOGGLES
SCRIBBLE
EXPLORE YOUR WEIRD FEELINGS
NOUS.CUBE@GMAIL.COM
* OF THE FUTURE PAST

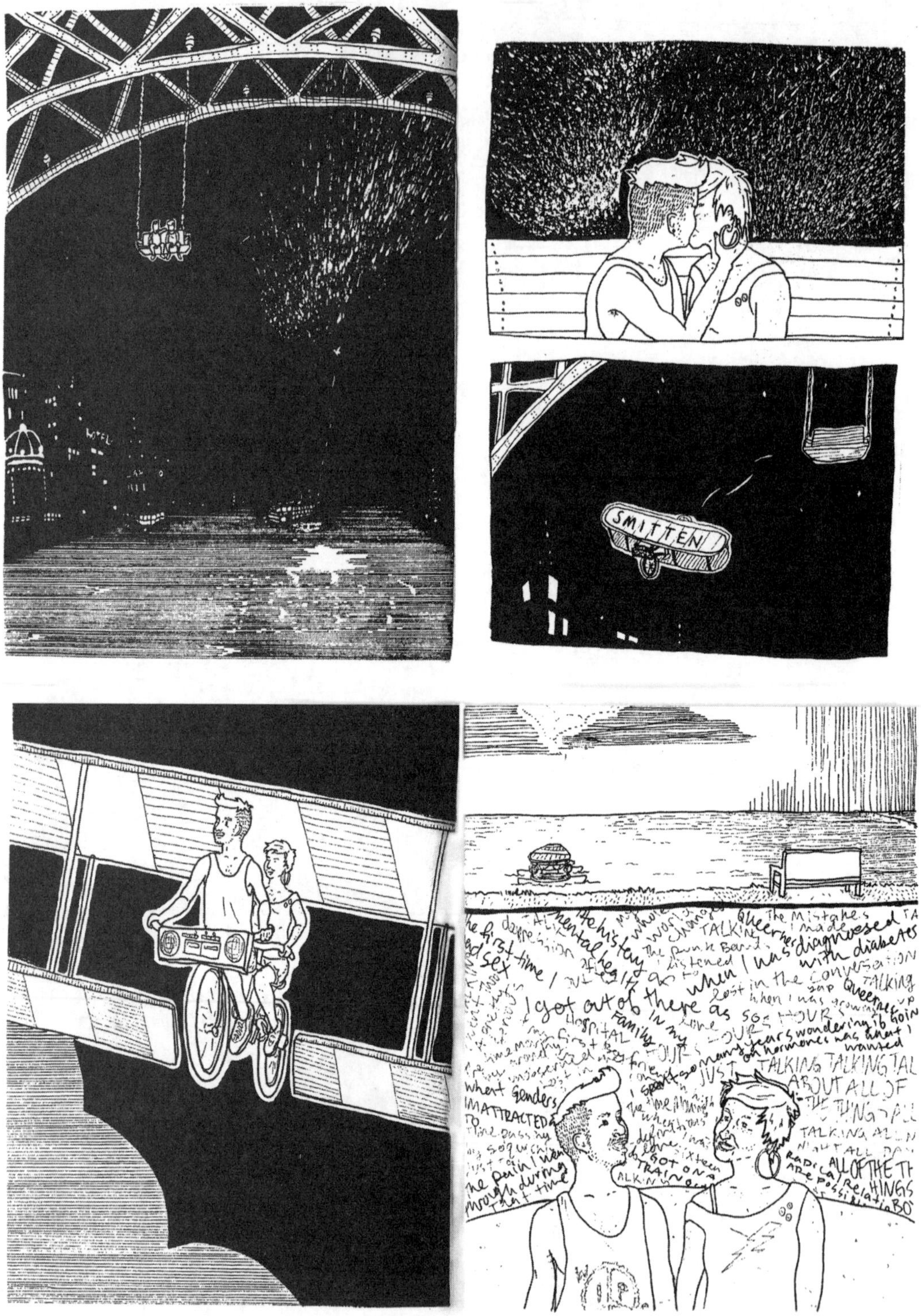
HOTEL
SMITTEN
mental health
the history
The Mistakes I made
Queerness
TALKING
The punk Band I listened to
when I was diagnosed with diabetes
lost in the conversation
I got out of there as
Family
HOSPITAL
so many years wondering if going on hormones was what I wanted
JUST
TALKING TALKING TAL
ABOUT ALL OF
What Genders I'M ATTRACTED TO
TALKING ALL NIGHT ALL DAY
ALL OF THE THINGS

BAH!
HEH
IM LEAVING TOWN FOR A WHILE
TAKE CARE OF THIS FOR ME?

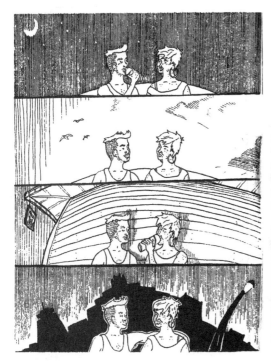

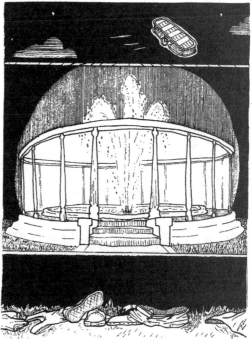

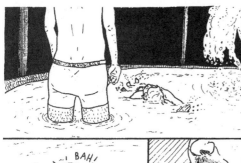

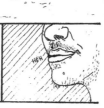

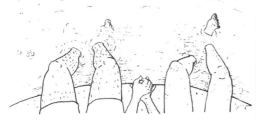

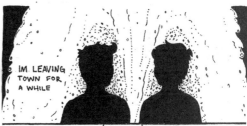

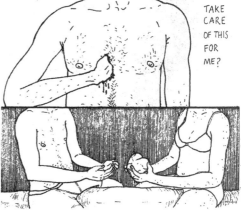

ABOUT THE EDITORS

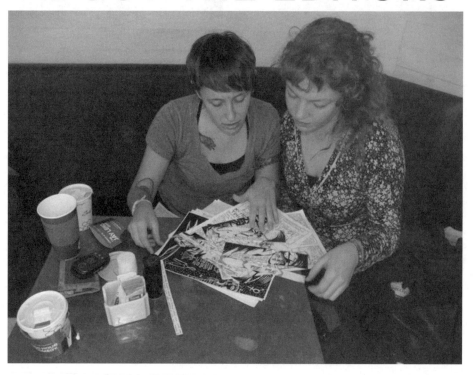

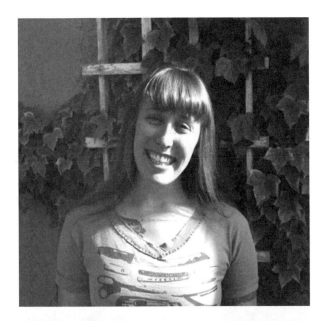

LIZA BLEY earned her BA from Eugene Lang College, The New School for Liberal Arts, where her senior project became the first incarnation of NYMM, and earned her MPH from the University of New Mexico. She contributed embroidery samples to the book *Embroider Everything Workshop* while working at Make, a craft and sewing school on the Lower East Side. Liza is committed to working with youth to improve the health of their communities.

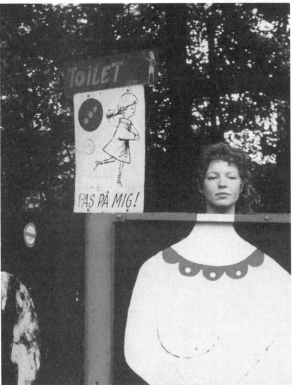

SAIYA MILLER graduated from Eugene Lang College, The New School for Liberal Arts with a BA in Culture and Media Studies. She has worked as an educator and activist, teaching art and music, as well as using comics and zines in workshops for teenagers. She currently lives in New Orleans.

ACKNOWLEDGMENTS

We would like to thank our families for their endless love and crucial input, our friends for their enthusiasm for the project since we started in 2008, Liz Parker, our editor, for her thoughtful comments and guidance, Emma Cofod for her graphic guidance, and everyone else at Soft Skull/Counterpoint Press, Erin Wilson for her keen eye and intuitive approach to the comics, The Comics and Medicine community for including us in an emerging genre, Ariel Schrag and Alison Bechdel for their support, each and every one of the contributors to the Not Your Mother's Meatloaf zines in the years before this book was put together, and the brave young people who shared their stories and inspired us at workshops and events along the way.

If you would like to see more of the following artists'
work, you can check it out at the sites listed below.

Grace Lang: gracelangillustration.com

Robnoxious: robnoxious.wordpress.com

Erin Wilson: The comic included is an excerpt from SNOWBIRD,
a webcomic that you can follow online at www.snowbirdcomic.com

Comic Nurse: www.comicnurse.com

Skip Heatwave: Facebook:
www.facebook.com/pages/SO-OUTTA-HERE/132884470074489
Blog: http:skipheatwave.blogspot.com

Sylvie le Sylvie: www.flickr.com/sylvieLS